Recognizing and Helping
the Neglected Child

Safeguarding Children Across Services
Series editors: Carolyn Davies and Harriet Ward

Safeguarding children from abuse is of paramount importance. This series communicates messages for practice from an extensive government-funded research programme designed to improve early recognition of child abuse as well as service responses and interventions. The series addresses a range of forms of abuse, including emotional and physical abuse and neglect, and outlines strategies for effective interagency collaboration, successful intervention and best practice. Titles in the series will be essential reading for practitioners with responsibility for safeguarding children.

Carolyn Davies is Research Advisor at Thomas Coram Research Unit at Institute of Education, University of London.

Harriet Ward is Director of the Centre for Child and Family Research and Research Professor at Loughborough University.

other books in the series

Safeguarding Children from Emotional Maltreatment
What Works
Jane Barlow and Anita Schrader McMillan
ISBN 978 1 84905 053 1

Caring for Abused and Neglected Children
Making the Right Decisions for Long-Term Care or Reunification
Jim Wade, Nina Biehal, Nicola Farrelly and Ian Sinclair
ISBN 978 1 84905 207 8

Adolescent Neglect
Research, Policy and Practice
Gwyther Rees, Mike Stein, Leslie Hicks and Sarah Gorin
ISBN 978 1 84905 104 0

Safeguarding Children Across Services
Messages from Research
Carolyn Davies and Harriet Ward
ISBN 978 1 84905 124 8

Safeguarding Children
Across Services

Recognizing and Helping the Neglected Child

Evidence-Based Practice for Assessment and Intervention

*Brigid Daniel, Julie Taylor and Jane Scott
with David Derbyshire and Deanna Neilson*

Foreword by Enid Hendry

Jessica Kingsley *Publishers*
London and Philadelphia

Figure 4.2 from Scottish Executive 2005 in Chapter 4 is reproduced by permission of the Controller of HMSO and the Queen's Printer for Scotland.

First published in 2011
by Jessica Kingsley Publishers
116 Pentonville Road
London N1 9JB, UK
and
400 Market Street, Suite 400
Philadelphia, PA 19106, USA

www.jkp.com

Library of Congress Cataloging in Publication Data
Recognizing and helping the neglected child : evidence-based practice for
assessment and intervention / Brigid Daniel ... [et al.] ; foreword by Enid
Hendry.
    p. cm.
  Includes bibliographical references and index.
  ISBN 978-1-84905-093-7 (alk. paper)
  1. Child welfare. 2. Child abuse. 3. Social work with children. 4.
Children--Services for. I. Daniel, Brigid, 1959-
  HV713.R434 2011
  362.76'532--dc23
                        2011021208

British Library Cataloguing in Publication Data
A CIP catalogue record for this book is available from the British Library

ISBN 978 1 84905 093 7

Printed and bound in Great Britain

Contents

List of Tables and Figures

Acknowledgements

The systematic literature that formed the basis for much of this book was funded by the Department of Health and the Department of Children, Schools and Families (now Department for Education) as part of the *Safeguarding Children Research Initiative.*

We are grateful to the practitioners who contributed the case study material that has helped us to illustrate the realities of practice with neglected children and provided a window into the creative and effective work that is being undertaken across the UK on behalf of neglected children.

We thank Mike Stein for permission to reproduce the material from Hicks and Stein (2010) as Tables 3.1 and 3.2.

The views expressed in this book are the authors' and do not necessarily reflect those of the Department of Health or the Department for Education.

Foreword

> Neglected children remain under the radar of professional awareness for too long, and outside the circle of protective intervention. (p.147)

The long-term effects of neglect are profoundly harmful and on far too many occasions fatal. While other forms of maltreatment appear to be reducing in frequency, the incidence of neglect has increased and now constitutes the majority of cases of significant harm. For practitioners it can be one of the most challenging, frustrating and dispiriting areas of practice. For all these reasons this book is a most welcome and timely addition to the literature on child neglect. The authors write with assurance and understanding, recognizing how emotionally draining and professionally demanding the work can be; they also offer a challenge to current thinking and practice.

This is a must-read book for all those whose work brings them in contact with neglected children, for their managers and those responsible for their training and education, for three main reasons. First it provides a succinct and authoritative synthesis of research, drawing on a systematic review of evidence on recognizing neglect. I found the distinction made between a broad definition of neglect and a narrow operational or professional definition of 'neglect' made sense, as did the authors' recommendation that, instead of getting unduly hung up on definitions, we should accept neglect as a fluid concept.

Second, the authors challenge the reader to reflect on their practice, values and ways of thinking about neglect and neglecting parents. I particularly like the authors' challenge to the notion of 'hard to reach' and 'hard to change' families, which they suggest we reframe in terms of 'hard to access' and 'hard to use' services. I was struck by their observation that the general public are at least as well equipped as professionals to recognize neglectful care, if not more so, and of the need to hear and act on the concerns of the wider community. They suggest it may not be that practitioners are failing to notice, rather that they are unsure or reluctant to act. There is a world of difference, they say, between noticing and responding.

Third, this is a book that empowers the reader. The authors re-affirm the importance of trusting intuition, of professional courage and of relationship. Key principles of effective intervention are identified, while they emphasize that 'who works' is as important as 'what works'. And finally the authors make a compelling case for a public health approach to tackling child neglect, which they argue offers the most coherent and systematic chance of success in preventing the flood of neglect cases that threatens to overwhelm the capacity of the child protection system. They argue persuasively that with early recognition and early response early in a child's life the appalling consequences of neglect can be prevented.

Enid Hendry
Head of Strategy and Development (Looked after Children), NSPCC

1

Understanding Child Neglect

Introduction

Neglect is, paradoxically, quite simple, but in many ways very complex. The simple and stark reality for children whose needs are not being met is that life is pretty miserable. For some children the neglect is so profound that they starve to death or die because of accidents associated with lack of supervision. And yet neglect appears to pose real challenges for researchers, theoreticians and national and local policy-makers. Much has been written about the difficulty of finding an agreed definition of neglect that would allow for more consistent research studies and findings that can be translated into practice in different settings. Much has also been written about the complexity of capturing the absence of something – that is – adequate physical and emotional care.

Neglect can be defined in terms of the impact upon the child or in terms of parental characteristics and behaviour, or both. Dubowitz *et al.* (1998) suggest that while specific developmental milestones that children need to reach are well established in child developmental theory, there is much less discussion or agreement about the minimum caregiving required in order to meet those milestones. Nor are there clear empirical standards for the parenting and conditions necessary for optimal child growth and development. Dubowitz *et al.* (2005) noted that neglect is difficult to define conceptually and operationally because it is a heterogeneous phenomenon, usually referring to complex situations and experienced differently by individual children. Neglect is often described on a continuum of care which ranges from excellent to grossly inadequate. It is easier to discern whether the care is meeting a child's needs at either end of the spectrum than in the middle.

For statutory systems neglect appears to continually pose challenges in the translation of concerns about children's unmet needs into action that enables those needs to be met and thus improves their lives.

Front-line practitioners from a range of disciplines often find themselves in an emotionally draining and dangerous middle territory in which they are simultaneously aware of the simple fact that a child needs help and the complex mechanism that has to be invoked in order to deliver help (see Figure 1.1).

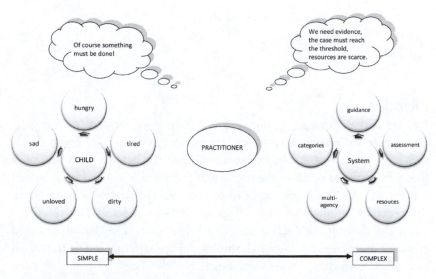

Figure 1.1: Showing the practitioner's dilemma when weighing up a child's need and system demands

Awareness of child neglect and its consequences on the future well-being and development of children has increased during the last two decades. During this time, considerable resources have been deployed to tackling the problem, but not always to best effect (Berry, Charlston and Dawson 2003; Scottish Executive 2002). The recognition of neglect is inconsistent and referrals to services are often triggered by other events or concerns about vulnerable children. In this book we provide practitioners with material that will be useful for practice with children whose needs are not being met for whatever reason. The core research evidence is drawn from our systematic review of the literature which is described in more detail later. One of the key conclusions from this review, though, was that there is still an absence of robust evidence in the field of neglect and so we have drawn on a wider range of literature including practice and policy material to develop the themes further.

Child neglect

The extent to which neglect can be considered a simple or complex phenomenon is evidenced by the range of approaches to definition. Horwath (2007) has helpfully collated many of these definitions and the resulting typology shows that they can range from a detailed breakdown of different forms of neglect to very broad definitions. Horwath, for example, identifies categories of neglect as:

- medical neglect
- nutritional neglect
- emotional neglect
- educational neglect
- physical neglect
- lack of supervision and guidance. (Horwath 2007, p.27)

English *et al.* (2005) start with a much broader definition couched in terms of unmet need:

> Neglect is defined in terms of child needs that are potentially unmet and subsequent impact on child functioning or development. (p.193)

There is a distinction to be drawn between neglect as a concept denoting the experience of a child whose developmental needs are not being met and 'neglect' as an operational, legislative or policy label. If one is wanting to understand the kind of caring environment that promotes happiness and health, then the concept of neglect can be a very broad one, but if one is developing a service with limited resources, or if one is applying some compulsory intervention 'neglect' can be a narrow category. A lot depends on what the definition is *for*. Definitions will be different depending on whether they are the basis for:

- criminal or civil legal proceedings
- national or local policy
- research on child development, aetiology, long-term outcomes
- research on the operation and effectiveness of practice
- determining eligibility for services

- delivering a service
- investigation of allegations
- rationing scarce resources.

For example, if a researcher is planning a study of neglect they will set the parameters of their study within a theoretical context. Depending on the theoretical standpoint and the research question the definition could be very broad or very narrow. A search for studies on neglect could throw up studies with research questions as contrasting as:

- What is the impact of material deprivation upon childhood educational attainment?

- What is the impact of maternal substance misuse upon the quality of the mother–child attachment relationships?

- Does child temperament affect response to emotional neglect?

- Is the state neglecting child asylum seekers?

- Which professionals attend case conferences called in relation to concerns about child neglect?

Although literature reviews often conclude with a plaintive plea for a common, international definition to enable comparison of research findings this is not a realistic goal because the territory of interest is so vast.

Of course, it is in the interests of equity, civil liberties and justice that there be some clear parameters when one moves closer to the terrain of state provision of services whether on a voluntary or compulsory basis, especially for action that could result in a child being removed from their family of origin. But, currently, when looking across the UK and at other jurisdictions with similar systems it is apparent that both broad and narrow definitions are operating simultaneously. There is a trend towards broad policy statements that draw attention to the importance of supporting children's developmental welfare and that especially emphasize the need for universal services to provide prompt support in the face of early signs of unmet need. There is a strong emphasis upon early intervention. For example, the emergent English and Scottish policy context has taken the wider ecological perspective on safeguarding and puts children's needs as the starting point (DFES 2004; Scottish Executive 2005). *Framework for the Assessment* (Department of Health 2000) is built around children's needs and again takes an ecological and developmental perspective. *The Children's Plan* (DCSF 2007a) clearly identifies the extent to which parenting is compromised by disadvantage and adversity and outlines strategies to provide timely support.

Such policies would, therefore, encompass broad definitions of neglect. When defining 'neglect' as a category for compulsory action, though, definitions become narrower. The operational definition of neglect for professional practice in England is:

> …the persistent failure to meet a child's basic physical and/or psychological needs, likely to result in the serious impairment of the child's health or development.
>
> Neglect may occur during pregnancy as a result of maternal substance abuse. Once a child is born, neglect may involve a parent or carer failing to:
>
> - provide adequate food, clothing and shelter (including exclusion from home or abandonment)
>
> - protect a child from physical and emotional harm or danger
>
> - ensure adequate supervision (including the use of inadequate care-givers)
>
> - ensure access to appropriate medical care or treatment.
>
> It may also include neglect of, or unresponsiveness to, a child's basic emotional needs. (HM Government 2010, p.12).

Framed in this way the definition appears very concrete – but all definitions are shaped by social factors, culture and values; for example, comparison with the previous definition shows that substance misuse during pregnancy is a recent addition, presumably in response to rises in referrals associated with substance misuse (Department of Health, Home Office and Department for Education and Employment 1999).

Although based in the evidence about factors that impact on child development the operational definition for England squarely locates 'neglect' as caregiver omission – unlike many research studies it does not locate the caregiver within a wider socio-economic context. The definition used for a wide-ranging literature review of incidence and prevalence of maltreatment in high-income countries (Gilbert *et al.* 2009) also takes a parent-focus (based on the Centers for Disease Control and Prevention report 2008 (Leeb *et al.* 2008)):

> Failure to meet a child's basic physical, emotional, medical/dental, or educational needs; failure to provide adequate nutrition, hygiene, or shelter; or failure to ensure a child's safety.

They add that this:

> includes failure to provide adequate food, clothing, or accommodation; not seeking medical attention when needed; allowing a child to miss large amounts of school; and failure to protect a child from violence in the home or neighbourhood or from avoidable hazards. Parents make up 87 per cent of perpetrators of substantiated cases in the USA. (p.168)

It is noticeable that these definitions are couched very much in terms of what parents are failing to do, and therefore chime with the notion of 'omission' which is often associated with definitions of neglect. The focus is on parental responsibility (and perhaps culpability) rather than upon children's needs and parenting is not overtly contextualized within wider social forces.

Again, it is front-line agencies and practitioners who have to navigate the choppy waters here. On the one hand it is vital that they keep hold of their broad understanding of children's needs and that their assessments are guided by sound developmental theory. One the other hand, access to services or delivery of services can be constrained by operational categories and labels. It is this tension that is often running below the almost constant discourse about thresholds. As seen in Figure 1.1, issues of 'thresholds' are a frequent source of anxiety. Buckley (2005) has depicted the problem as an egg-timer where there are needs that are perceived to have to be squeezed through a narrow isthmus to get at the services below – and the isthmus is guarded by statutory child protection processes. Policies are trying to shift us towards a different model where all agencies are seen as part of one system with a range of services. The aspiration is that access to services should not depend on attaining a system label – in this instance 'neglect' and that there should not be a concept of moving the child from 'outside' to 'inside' a system to get a service. The extent to which this aspiration can be attained, especially as resources are limited is still open to question, but we would suggest that the 'longing for clear thresholds' as Stevenson puts it (2007, p.7) is as vain as the search for one settled definition. In effect the threshold is really the space between neglect and 'neglect' and somehow practitioners have to simultaneously keep hold of both broad and narrow definitions.

Interestingly, in Scotland, it is proposed to remove the requirement to identify a category of concern when placing a child's name on the child protection register and instead to do so only:

where there are reasonable grounds to believe or suspect that a child has suffered or will suffer significant harm from abuse or neglect, and that a Child Protection Plan is needed to protect and support the child. (Scottish Government 2010a, p.18)

Definitions of different forms of maltreatment are still provided and it is required to set out the areas of risk that the plan will address. This proposal tackles the fact that different forms of abuse and neglect often coincide, and may help address the problem of trying to fit the particular circumstances of an individual child into a specific 'box'.

Another issue that needs to be considered when defining neglect is chronicity. Classically, neglect is noted for its chronic nature. In relation to ongoing child development and well-being it is the chronic nature of neglect that is known to be particularly corrosive. However, the protective systems, like those in England, that have developed around a forensic core, are notoriously clumsy when it comes to dealing with sustained problems rather than one-off events. This is increasingly being acknowledged and recognized. For example, in Victoria, Australia, the state government has incorporated the concept of 'cumulative harm' into the Children, Youth and Families Act 2005. One of the underlying principles of the act is that it is necessary to consider 'the effects of cumulative patterns of harm on a child's safety and development' (s. 10(3)(e)). Cumulative harm has to be considered in relation to all forms of maltreatment, but it is noted that it is most likely to be pertinent in situations of neglect. Bromfield and Miller (2007) define it thus:

> Cumulative harm refers to the effects of multiple adverse circumstances and events in a child's life. The unremitting daily impact of these experiences on the child can be profound and exponential, and diminish a child's sense of safety, stability and wellbeing.
>
> Cumulative harm may be caused by an accumulation of a single recurring adverse circumstance or event (e.g., unrelenting low level care), or by multiple different circumstances and events (e.g., persistent verbal abuse and denigration, inconsistent or harsh discipline and/or exposure to family violence). (p.1)

While legislation in other jurisdictions may not incorporate cumulative harm in this overt manner, the concept is a very helpful one for defining an accumulation of deleterious effects upon a child's development.

At the same time, though, context can be an important factor because it is possible to define one-off lapses of supervision or care, even if unintended, as 'neglect' and, indeed, single incidents can be highly dangerous or fatal, for example, a parent forgetting to shut the front door so that a young child walks into the road. Practitioners in family support, children and families social services or teaching are not routinely expected to be providing services in relation to such one-off manifestations of lack of supervision and which tend not to be defined as 'neglect'. But the *prevention* of such incidents could well be seen as falling in the province of some professionals, for example, health visitors who advise parents about young children's capacity; the police who are involved in accident prevention and local councillors and planners who must consider issues of road safety, traffic calming and child safety. Horwath (2007) discusses the huge difficulties entailed in distinguishing between true accidents and accidents resulting from neglect and we return to this issue in Chapter 3.

Rather than trying to pin down neglect we would suggest that it is better to accept that it is a fluid concept. We have to avoid allowing our system categories, that have been developed for very specific purposes, driving our wider perceptions and assessments of what children need. A definition must be the key not the padlock. At the same time, practitioners must be aware of the legislative framework within which they work and the important safeguards they aim to provide, even if the balance can be tricky at times. Legislation, in most jurisdictions, is trying to support a careful balance between allowing the capacity to intervene on behalf of children, and the protection of the integrity of their family life and their parents' rights to parent in their own way. Practitioners need to work within the spirit of these aspirations while avoiding becoming so preoccupied with bureaucratic demands that they forget the point of their work in the first place. It may have become a cliché, but it really is vital to keep *the child at the centre* of practice. This does not mean riding rough-shod over the wishes and needs of parents or ignoring their rights – it is not in children's best interests to undermine their parents. But it does mean keeping a determined focus on whether the child is receiving an acceptable level of care, and if they are not, thinking about what would make a difference for them and making sure something is done (see Box 1.1).

Box 1.1 Activity

We suggest that the straightforward aim of providing help to children whose needs are not being met has become obscured within the complexities of our formal helping systems. Legislation, policy and guidance have developed with good intentions, but have shaped into a particularly unwieldy practice framework for neglect. We can lose sight of children and their needs in the clutter of bureaucratic systems and language. An unhappy child is hidden within a thicket of jargon such as 'referral', 'report', 'recognition', 'initial enquiry', 'threshold', 'investigation', 'response', 'evidence', 'assessment', 'planning', 'intervention', 'monitoring', 'package of care', 'protection plan', 'review', 'outcome'.

Instead it may be helpful to return to some very simple concepts that spring from the child's perspective. From the child's point of view there are three fundamental issues:

- what I need to grow and develop
- what I need people to think about
- what I need people to do.

1. Thinking about a child who you are concerned about, consider the following questions and note down your thoughts. Try to step back from the system within which you operate and avoid using the language of bureaucracy or jargon or 'shorthand' terms:

   a. What does this child need to grow and develop and what does their family or carer need to provide a nurturing environment?

   b. What does this child and their family or carer need me to think about?

   c. What does this child and their family or carer need me to do?

2. Note how well you were able to curb the use of jargon and system terminology.

3. Think about how you can translate the answers to these three key questions into the language of the system within which you are required to operate to make sure that the child gets the help they need.

Recognition and response

Much emphasis is placed upon awareness-raising to improve practice with neglect and the term 'recognition and response' is frequently used as if the two are one and the same. But, in reality, there is a world of difference between recognizing and responding – the first is relatively simple, the second is far more complex. It is certainly important to improve both recognition and response, and there are close connections between them, but we suggest that it is helpful to consider each process separately and to look at the different factors that affect them. Therefore, in the first part of this book we focus on recognition and in the latter part move onto detailed consideration of response.

Recognizing

Recognizing the structural and parental factors associated with neglect is not that complicated if seen in a fairly commonsense way. Practitioners encountering adults who misuse substances, are living with domestic violence or have mental health problems can, with only a little reflection, recognize the likely impact upon children. Housing officers who are called to deal with chaotic and dirty households can easily imagine what it must be like for children to live in these conditions. Police officers attending domestic abuse incidents encounter distressed children. Many practitioners also recognize neglected children, even if they do not label them thus – they are children who are dirty, unkempt, miss school, under-perform in school, have few friends, are either underfed or obese, miss health checks and appointments and, above all, are often sad and lonely. For many members of extended families, people in the community and other children, it is also not difficult to identify such children. There are also many more subtle indications of neglect that can be recognized with careful attention and assessment.

Chapters 2 and 3 cover recognition in more detail. Chapter 2 explores the evidence about the factors that affect parenting, ranging from structural stresses to individual personal issues, and how they may be manifested and identified. It also considers the evidence about ways in which parents may directly and indirectly signal that they are struggling to provide sufficient care for their children. Chapter 3 reviews the research about the obvious and less obvious signs that a child's developmental needs are not being met to the extent that well-being is, or is likely to be compromised. The ways in which children may signal their need for help and the factors that make it difficult to seek help on their own behalf are examined. Together, these chapters show that there is no lack of potential signs and signals that a child's needs may be unmet. This information should support the practitioner with the question:

- What does this child need to grow and develop and what does their family or carer need to provide a nurturing environment?

Responding

There are, however, gaps between:

- the existence of such signs and signals

- someone first recognizing them as indicators of a form of child maltreatment that might merit intervention, and

- then knowing how best to respond.

Many practitioners describe the high levels of anxiety they feel about such children: teachers describe sleepless nights wondering what they should do; health visitors talk of their frustration in trying to make referrals to social services. There appear to be all sorts of barriers in place that prevent swift provision of help to neglected children. They include issues of role definition, confidence, hierarchies and status, procedures and bureaucracy, resources, working relationships with families and many more. It is likely that, for some people, the only way to reduce some of the anxiety about such children is to cease recognizing the problem in the first place. The difficulty of knowing how best to help can help to create a 'neglect-filter' which enables neglect to be screened out with thoughts such as 'it's not that bad really', 'they're happy underneath it', 'I've seen worse'. Some of these screening out processes have become so routine that they operate as received wisdom voiced in phrases such as 'children can be dirty but happy'; 'people who misuse substances can be perfectly good parents'; 'it is wrong to impose middle-class values on poor parents' and so on.

Effective practice is often hampered by practitioner anxiety about making value judgements and about being judgemental. Practitioners need to be able to distinguish being between judgemental and making well-evidenced, ethical *professional judgements* on behalf of children. They need to consider issues of physical, emotional, educational, medical and cognitive neglect and to begin to explore relative thresholds and the impact of different professional cultures. They also need to guard against cultural relativism and the fear of making racist judgements – an issue that was highly relevant to decisions in relation to Victoria Climbié (Lord Laming 2003).

The effect of context and the difference between neglect and 'neglect' can be illustrated by the research on the ways different people perceive and define neglect. In particular, it appears that the general public see neglect rather than 'neglect' – their views are not affected by thinking about system categories, thresholds or service provision. Rather they see a child they are worried about and think something should be done. In this regard their perceptions are akin to the 'simple' element in Figure 1.1. In a series of studies Rose and colleagues compared the views of the general public with those of professionals. They asked respondents to rate a series of one-line statements relating to the adequacy of care of a six-year-old child. In the States the responses of mothers were compared with child protection investigators and case workers (Rose and Meezan 1995, 1996). The statements tended to cluster into four main factors and there was general agreement that behaviour such as not offering a six-year-old child food at a fixed time each day; leaving the child alone outside after dark; not taking the child to a doctor when ill, were likely to cause the child harm. Overall, the mothers gave higher ratings of seriousness than the case workers. A smaller study in England also found that a group of mothers consistently rated statements exemplifying lack of care as more serious that a group of social workers (Rose and Selwyn 2000). In a similar study in the US Dubowitz *et al.* (1998) found that members of the community expressed higher levels of concern than child maltreatment professionals. It could be argued that practitioners are more concerned about recognizing 'neglect' than neglect.

Such research also helps us to understand why official prevalence figures are lower than might be expected. State figures are drawn from official statistics about child protection proceedings and whether children are the subject of child protection plans. But this, of course, marks the culmination of a significant filtering process and such statistics are measuring 'neglect' as an operational category. Even by these figures neglect tends to be the most frequent category of maltreatment to be referred (reported) in high income countries (Gilbert *et al.* 2009). Studies of prevalence, such as that by May-Chahal and Cawson (2005), as described in Box 1.2, are likely to give a more reliable picture of children's actual experiences than official 'child protection' statistics. They found that not only is prevalence higher than reported figures suggest, but that people tend not to label their own experiences as abusive.

Box 1.2 Research highlight

May-Chahal, C., and Cawson, P. (2005) 'Measuring child maltreatment in the United Kingdom: A study of the prevalence of child abuse and neglect.' *Child Abuse and Neglect, 29*, 9, 969–984.

The overall aim of this NSPCC-funded study was to obtain a profile of the prevalence of abuse and neglect in the UK child population by asking young people aged between 18 and 24 to reflect on their childhood experiences. However, with the knowledge that people tend not to describe themselves as having been maltreated, the methodology was designed to collect both descriptive data about actual childhood experiences of positive and negative treatment and separate subjective judgements from respondents about whether they considered any of the treatment they received to have been child abuse.

A series of treatments was set out in a questionnaire and 2896 respondents noted whether they had experienced them, and if so in what context and how seriously. At the end of each section they were asked to note whether they considered the treatment to have been child abuse.

For the purposes of this study neglect was defined as 'lack of physical care and lack of supervision' (p.972) and a set of criteria used to define it as 'serious', 'intermittent' or 'a cause for concern'. The criteria used for 'serious' neglect were based on evidence about features likely to cause harm and therefore may be useful also for practice assessments – *serious* absence of care criteria included:

- Aged <12 always/often went hungry because no one got your meals ready or there was no food in the house.
- Aged <12 always/often were ill but no one looked after you or took you to the doctors.
- Aged <12 always/often went to school in dirty clothes because there were no clean ones available.
- Often had to look after themselves because parents had problems, for example, alcohol or drugs.
- Regularly had to look after self because parents went away.
- Allowed to go into dangerous places or situations.
- Abandoned or deserted.
- Physical condition of their home was dangerous. (p.974)

Serious lack of supervision entailed:

> ...children were allowed to stay at home unsupervised under the age of 10 or allowed to stay out overnight without parents knowing their whereabouts under the age of 14. (pp.972–973)

Over 90 per cent agreed that they had a 'warm and loving family background' (p.976). Fifteen per cent said they regularly had to look after themselves because of parental problems such as substance misuse or because parents went away. Four per cent regularly had to help care for someone in the family who was ill or disabled.

Only 2 per cent of the respondents rated themselves as having been neglected. However, from the description of the treatment they received, 6 per cent were gauged to have experienced a serious absence of care; 9 per cent an intermediate lack of care and 2 per cent an absence of care that was a cause for concern. Five per cent were judged to have experienced a serious lack of supervision and 12 per cent an intermediate lack of supervision.

The authors conclude 'this research has found that young people could experience severe lack of care, physical violence, or sexual abuse and not rate themselves as abused. In addition very few people reported their abuse to the authorities' (p.982).

In Chapter 4 we set out the evidence from our review of studies that have considered recognition and response by the general public and practitioners. We suggest that people first need to feel confident about their intuitions and concerns about what they are seeing and then need to be clear about what to do next but that many things can affect such confidence and clarity. This process of taking stock of what is being seen and then deciding what to do about it should be an iterative process and should continue on a longer-term basis. In essence this is what good assessment and planning entails. There are a number of existing books that address the issue of assessment of neglect in detail so we do not aim to duplicate them here (Department of Health 1999; Horwath 2001, 2007; Stevenson 2007; Taylor and Daniel 2005). However, in Chapter 4 we also consider some of the issues associated specifically with the process of assessing the meaning of the observed signs that parents and children may need help, and planning what can be done to make the child's life better.

Much like the term 'recognition and response' the term 'assessment and planning' can mask the differences between these two different stages of activity. We have previously suggested that anxiety about how best to intervene on behalf of a child can interfere with careful assessment of the ways in which that child's needs are not being met and why (Daniel 2005). We reiterate that message here. First it is essential to delineate the ways in which the child's needs are not being met and the current and likely future effect on the child. All anxieties and concerns about the solution should be set aside at this stage. Instead of tussling over who should do what and who should pay for what, the professionals and para-professionals involved should galvanize their activities around:

- assessing the child's unmet needs in all domains
- assessing the reasons for needs not being met
- assessing parental capacity to meet those needs
- assessing parental motivation to meet the child's needs with support
- assessing parental capacity to adapt and change with support.

It is only possible to develop a sensible plan for improving the child's life once all the information about what is going wrong has been brought together and made sense of. In other words, there needs to be a proper assessment which is then followed by a plan of action.

In practice, though, 'assessment' as an official activity seems to have become laden with complexity and anxiety, especially in the UK. It has become associated with bureaucratic demands, complicated computer-based systems, pressure of timescales and fears about risk. We suggest that, in fact, assessment need not be so complicated and anxiety-laden. There is plenty of research evidence and theory to help with understanding children's developmental needs and parental capacity to meet them. Such evidence is now incorporated into the frameworks for assessment used in many countries. Certainly, there are logistical challenges, especially when different professionals hold different bits of information which need to be collated. Certainly, also, it takes time and thought to undertake a proper analysis of all the information. But it takes a lot more time and resource to undo the damage of precipitous action.

Brandon *et al.* (2008) persuasively argue that an ecological-transactional-developmental framework provides the most helpful theoretical framework for understanding and assessing children's needs and parental capacity to meet them. We would agree that this theoretical approach is currently one of the most helpful for assessment and planning in relation to neglect – but it does entail a daunting array of factors to consider in relation to each individual child. There are no quick assessment shortcuts.

Another pitfall is the tendency towards 'assessment paralysis' (Reder and Lucey 1995) which can lead to constant assessment and re-assessment and no planning and action. Practitioners therefore need to understand the difference between collation and analysis of information, and build on the assessment framework in use in their jurisdiction (for example, Department of Health 2000). Practitioners need to be able to distinguish between:

- an assessment of a child's needs and where they are unmet

- an assessment of the reason for the needs being unmet, and

- an assessment about whether compulsory measures might be required and develop plans accordingly.

Once the information has been brought together planning entails deciding who will do what, when and how to ensure that the child's needs are met. Based on the assessment of parental capacity and motivation to change within appropriate timescales the plan should propose a proportionate level of legislative compulsion, which, if proved wrong should be amended accordingly. Although practitioners make many decisions they often fail to take decisions and follow them through in a sustained way. Planning has to involve consideration of different options and routes to effective intervention and must involve children and families – in particular, the involvement of children and young people in planning can be linked with improving their sense of self-efficacy – key to the development of resilience. Because neglect affects so many aspects of children's development, plans should facilitate each profession to deliver their core service to children whatever the level of parental capacity. The plan should therefore set out what will be done to ensure that the child has proper access to the universal services of education, health and leisure – a theme that we cover in more detail in Chapter 4. All this can be summed up from the child's perspective as:

- What does this child and their family or carer need me to think about?

Intervention

In Chapter 5 we consider what can be done to improve the child's life. For too many neglected children intervention does not lead to an appreciable improvement in their day-to-day lives; often this is the case even if a number of professionals do become involved. In some cases intervention leads to children experiencing even more disruption, fractured attachments, uncertain futures and fragmented services. The reasons for this are many and include:

- the complex nature of neglect and its aetiology
- the complex interaction of structural disadvantages, poverty, racism and poor housing, with parental circumstances and characteristics
- the range of different personal, cultural and professional values about what constitutes good enough parenting and good enough developmental progress
- professional paralysis in the face of what appear to be intractable and overwhelming circumstances
- intra- and inter-organizational bureaucratic structures that mitigate against flexible, tailored, creative and responsive action on behalf of children.

There is also a lack of sufficient rigorous empirical research into effective intervention, especially as provided by teachers, health professionals and the police.

What little evidence there is about effective intervention with neglect points to the need to build comprehensive packages of support that are clear, focused and address the issues at each ecological level (Berry *et al.* 2003). In particular there is evidence that the provision of direct support for children is of especial value (Gaudin 1993b). Despite the prevalent discourse, lack of resources is often not the main problem in cases of neglect – all too often children and families are bombarded with services that appear to have little appreciable impact on the quality of the child's day-to-day life (Scottish Executive 2002). Therefore, intervention has to include attention to the *processes* underlying service use and change. In particular, effective intervention can hinge on the quality of the relationship between practitioner and parent and or child (Barlow with Scott 2010).

Two syndromes are especially prevalent in practice with neglect, the 'rule of optimism' (Dingwall, Eekelaar and Murray 1995) and the 'start-again' syndrome (Brandon *et al.* 2008). At their extreme they can be fatal for children. The problem is often compounded when parents and carers appear to be complying with plans or when parents and carers deflect practitioner attention from the needs of children (Reder and Duncan 1995; Reder, Duncan and Gray 1993). In Chapter 5 we encourage readers to maintain a sharp focus on the extent to which children's lives are improved and whether the pace of change is in tune with children's rate of development. Effective reviewing of the impact of intervention has to be based upon determined, sustained and effective intervention to improve children's lives. The aim is to equip practitioners with a solid knowledge base and the confidence to put that knowledge into practice on behalf of children. Chapter 5 is informed by a literature review (Moran 2009) and a study of intervention (details at www.actionforchildren.org.uk/uploads/media/36/8092.pdf) both undertaken with Action for Children. In summary this chapter aims to help practitioners answer the question:

- What does this child and their family or carer need me to do?

The case study in Box 1.3 brings this set of questions together.

Box 1.3 Case study

Stacey (10) is of White British ethnicity. Her mother, Angela (39), unemployed, is from Northern Ireland but spent most of her childhood living in England. Stacey has no contact with her biological father who is currently incarcerated for sexually abusing Stacey's older sibling. Stacey has three sisters all of whom have different fathers, Lisa (16), Sarah (5) and Leah (3). The family lives in a five bedroom, rented bungalow in a small village on the outskirts of town. Stacey has regular contact with her maternal extended family who live nearby. Stacey's mother is in receipt of state benefits and receives no additional financial support from Stacey's father.

When the project worker, Sally, calls to collect Stacey for the afterschool sports club, Stacey opens the door and there is a strong smell of stale rubbish and bin bags of overflowing rubbish are observed lying in the hallway. Stacey is agitated that she is not ready to leave yet and asks Sally to wait while she searches for something appropriate to wear. Stacey calls out to her mother for help to find a tracksuit and t-shirt, her mother does not appear but is heard calling to Stacey to hurry up. Stacey runs to and from rooms looking for something to wear as well as looking through piles of clothes which are lying in the hallway next to the rubbish. Stacey calls Sally into the hallway to wait and Sally observes dirty cups, glasses, plates, dirty nappies and rubbish and there is a strong unpleasant odour. When Stacey emerges from her bedroom, her clothes appear dirty and ill-fitting. Sally calls to her mother who shouts back that she can't come out because one of the children has fallen asleep on her knee. Stacey and Sally leave, Stacey calls goodbye but there is no response from Mum.

Emotional interaction and physical affection between Stacey and her mother are infrequent and poor. Consequently, Stacey

---

has been observed to seek affection and individual attention from other children her own age, older children and adults. Much of this attention is physical such as hugs and kisses. Not only does this make Stacey extremely vulnerable, it also affects her relationships with her peers and her ability to maintain friendships. It is widely documented that children who do not receive sufficient emotional support from a parent will seek this elsewhere and this vulnerability can place children at considerable risk.

When the group arrive at the sports hall, Stacey runs up to hug the facilitators and throughout the session leaves the group to seek physical attention and conversation from staff members. At one point Stacey leaves the activity and shares with staff that she is uncomfortable because her t-shirt is too small and keeps riding up and exposing her tummy. Stacey is overweight and self-conscious about her stomach. Due to her level of discomfort and self-consciousness, Stacey chose not to participate in the activity and sat on the sidelines for the remainder of the session.

At the end of the session, Sally talked to Stacey about her experience of coming to the group that day. Sally made Stacey aware that she had noticed her difficulties at getting ready for the group and discomfort with her clothing. Sally advised that she would talk to her mother about this with a view to Stacey's needs being better met in future.

Early intervention and prevention

Even if we perfect our interventions children will still have experienced neglect – we, therefore, also need to look at policy and practice to prevent children suffering in the first place. As indicated above, policy in many jurisdictions has been steadily moving towards a model of earlier intervention, both in relation to age, but also in the stage of the problem. The vision of an integrated approach for children's services is at the heart of government policy (DCSF 2007a; Department of Health 1999, 2004; Department of Health, Home Office and DFES 2003; DFES 2004; HM Government 2010). Integrated approaches should be responsive to children's needs, proportionate and offered on a continuum: universal support for all parents and children; targeted support for those at risk of not achieving their potential; and responsive intervention on behalf of children with urgent needs for protection (DCSF 2007b). It is important to identify as early as possible children experiencing disadvantage such as incipient neglect and to deliver services that will prevent harm. In Chapter 6 we will draw the messages together and consider how they can help shape a swifter response to children who may need some additional support.

However, earlier intervention is *still* some steps away from prevention on a broader level. The prevalence of child maltreatment has led to it being increasingly conceptualized as a public health issue that can be tackled by tried and tested public health approaches. These entail dealing with causal social and cultural factors on a population-wide basis in order to lower rates of the issue of concern. There is an emerging consensus that we now know enough about the factors that contribute to neglect to be able to make some significant impact at population level. Whether neglect can be totally eradicated is questionable, but we argue in Chapter 6 that the kind of policies that would benefit potentially neglected children would also benefit all children. As Horton (2003) observes:

> Maltreatment is one of the biggest paediatric public-health challenges, yet any research activity is dwarfed by work on more established childhood ills… As with any other clinical problem, that of child maltreatment requires the development of a comprehensive research agenda to inform and improve prevention, diagnosis, interventions, and public-health provisions. Without such commitment, the true scandal is not the failure of a handful of individual professionals in notorious cases, but the systematic failure of all relevant professions towards the generations of children at risk to come. (p.443)

The research study

Our systematic review of the literature examined the published research evidence on the extent to which practitioners are equipped to recognize and respond to the indications that a child's needs are likely to be, or are being neglected, whatever the cause. It considered evidence about the ways in which children and families signal their need for help, how those signals are recognized and responded to and whether response could be swifter. The aim was to contribute to the evidence base that equips:

- practitioners with the information they need to be able and willing to recognize that a child's needs are not being met, or are in danger of being unmet, and consider themselves to be part of a protective network around children

- organizations with the information they need to ensure that their services are easily accessible to children and parents who need support and help

- policy-makers who make recommendations to the health, education and social care sectors regarding the needs of and response to neglected children

- education and training bodies, both statutory and voluntary, who provide access to and information about the evidence to relevant individuals.

The research questions were:

1. What is known about the ways in which children and families directly and indirectly signal their need for help?

2. To what extent are practitioners equipped to recognize and respond to the indications that a child's needs are likely to be, or are being neglected, whatever the cause?

3. Does the evidence suggest that professional response could be swifter?

In keeping with the themes we introduced earlier, when undertaking an international review the number of potential definitions of neglect becomes even wider. To keep the study as inclusive as possible, therefore, we did not set out a specific definition of neglect and kept as broad a definition as possible that was centred on the concept of unmet developmental need. Following a rigorous process of establishing the quality and relevance of published material, 63 papers, describing empirical studies undertaken in various parts of the world were included in the final review (see Appendix 1 for details of the methodology).

The analysis of included studies showed that definitions of neglect are slippery. The strongly rated studies provide good models for the development of further research. The limitations in the research were that studies tended to be mono-disciplinary, to be preoccupied with professional issues and formal protective systems, to use a wide range of proxy measures and case records and to conflate neglect and abuse.

Figure 1.2 shows the breakdown of included studies by the primary ecological focus (allowing for overlap between studies). The evidence-base for the first question, addressed in Chapters 2 and 3, is largely provided from studies dealing with child, family and social characteristics. The second and third questions, covered mainly in Chapter 4, are addressed primarily from the largest single group of studies, those that focused on professional issues. We also draw on other literature, especially in Chapters 5 and 6.

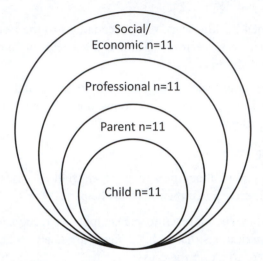

Figure 1.2: Showing the number of studies addressing factors at different ecological levels (allowing for some overlap between studies)

As shown in Figure 1.3, the greater proportion of studies on professional issues related to the health profession (allowing for overlap between studies).

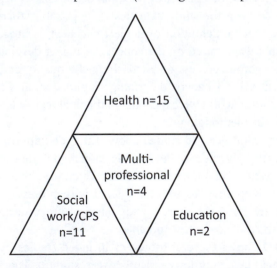

Figure 1.3: Showing the numbers of studies focusing on each profession, from the group of studies that focused mainly on professional issues (allowing for some overlap between studies)

When interpreting the evidence from this review it is important to take account of the limitations of this study. Any filtering process entails discarding potentially valuable evidence. In many studies the focus is on 'maltreatment' more broadly which means that different forms of neglect and abuse are conflated and that findings cannot be linked specifically to neglect only. We were broadly inclusive because we were aware that much of the evidence was likely to emerge from a broad range of research designs including qualitative studies. However, the risk of using a broad filter is that studies can be included that have limits of validity, reliability and generalizability. Some of the challenges of methodology mirror challenges in practice. The dilemma about whether to focus on parent behaviour, child outcomes or a mixture of both is shared between research and practice. Across all the studies a vast range of standardized, customized and proxy measures was employed, indicating the breadth and complexity of neglect and its antecedents. The preoccupation with substantiated neglect and with system processes also mirrors practitioner experience. So we have tried not to stretch the evidence too far in this book.

Much of the evidence collated was collected in countries other than the UK, including Europe and, most commonly, the US. This raises questions about the extent to which the lessons are transferable across countries. Our view is that the evidence drawn from studies focusing specifically on systems should be transferred with more caution than the evidence that focuses more on parenting capacity and children's development and we have borne this in mind in this book.

Overall, though, the review highlighted some of the huge gaps in the evidence-base to support practice. It is, therefore, not surprising that professionals are often relying heavily on practice wisdom. It is our view that, while there is now a large amount of research that confirms the negative impact of neglect upon children, there is a need for much research on how best to prevent neglect, support children who are at risk of being neglected and deal with neglect quickly.

KEY MESSAGES

1. In some ways child neglect is not a complicated concept when considered from the child's perspective, but the need to respond within the legislative and organizational context adds a number of layers of complexity.
2. Practitioner anxiety in the face of complexity could be alleviated if neglect is expected to be a multifaceted phenomenon.

3. There are a range of different definitions which can vary depending on their purpose. They can be broad and begin from children's unmet needs, or narrower and focus more on parental omission.

4. As policy develops over the next few years there may be merit in framing a definition of neglect based on an ecological-transactional-developmental model that includes reference to children's developmental needs, caregiver characteristics and socio-economic factors.

5. Recognizing that a child's needs are not being, or may not be met entails noticing the direct and indirect signs in the child and the factors that may be affecting parental capacity. The general population and practitioners in an array of professions have the potential to spot these signs without requiring specialist knowledge of child development.

6. A number of factors can affect the choices practitioners make about how to respond to signs of potential neglect. The discourse about social service 'thresholds' springs, in part, from systems and processes and can impede effective response to children.

7. Effective planning to help children depends on comprehensive assessment that draws on the knowledge and skills of all key professions and that pays close attention to the needs that are not being met and analyses why.

8. When services are provided to help children and families it is vital to monitor whether they are, in fact, making the child's life better.

9. Given its prevalence and the levels of harm to children, there is a lot of promise in taking a public-health approach to neglect which tackles the precipitating factors on a population-wide basis.

10. There is a need for more robustly designed, prospective, multi-disciplinary studies that move beyond a focus on formal systems towards a focus on the early indications of emergent neglect.

2

Signs that Parents Need Support

Introduction

Parenting, while often rewarding, can be challenging, demanding and worrying. All parents draw on various types of informal help from friends and family; many parents draw on various types of formal help from a range of services. Even under the best of circumstances things can happen that temporarily affect the quality of care that is provided to children. The backdrop, therefore, to all practice should be the assumption that anyone who is a parent could, at any time, need a bit of help – practical, emotional or both. As suggested in Chapter 1, the question to be asked is:

- What does this child's family or carer need to provide a nurturing environment?

Not everyone, though, who needs it, actually either asks for help, or gets help. There can be different reasons for this: some people do not really recognize that they need help, others find it hard to articulate either to themselves or others that they are struggling, some people think that they should be able to manage, others that they do not deserve support from others. Informal help from friends and family is often offered spontaneously, or is part of a reciprocal web of support. In the absence of mutual support, having to ask directly for help is frightening, and can feel demeaning. In relation to services provided by the independent, voluntary or state sectors the issues become more complex because parents are then reaching across the family-state boundary. Even the take-up of broad-based family support services (such as Sure Start in England) is not without its complications, but as one comes closer to situations that might be defined as 'neglect', issues of support can become affected by the backdrop of child protection preoccupations.

It cannot, therefore, be assumed that parents whose children are, or might be neglected, will identify themselves and directly ask for help. There is some evidence to assist with understanding direct help-seeking which is discussed later in the chapter. However, neglected children will be overlooked unless practitioners are alert to the more indirect signals that support is needed. These signals relate to factors that affect parenting such as substance misuse, mental health problems and domestic abuse. In order to be effective in recognizing potential neglect practitioners need a greater understanding of the ways in which such factors can affect parenting and the ways in which their effects are manifested by parents.

Factors associated with neglect

The more practitioners know about the factors that can affect parenting capacity to the extent that children's development may be compromised, the better they are equipped to recognize situations where there may be a need for more help. In short, practitioners should be able to recognize aspects of parental behaviour that can reasonably be expected to impact on children.

The studies in this review confirm existing evidence that mothers who neglect often have:

- mental health problems (Carter and Myers 2007; Cash and Wilke 2003; Sheehan 2004)

- low self-esteem (Cash and Wilke 2003)

- fewer problem-solving skills (Coohey 1998)

- fewer parenting skills, poorer knowledge of parenting and child development; poorer connection and less empathy with their children

- a history of abuse in childhood (Connell-Carrick and Scannapieco 2006; Scannapieco and Connell-Carrick 2005)

- a history of substance misuse (Jaudes, Ekwo and VanVoorhis 1995; McKeganey, Barnard and McIntosh 2002), and are parenting alone (Hultman et al. 1998; Thyen et al. 1997).

However, our systematic review of research about ways in which parents signal their need for help confirmed that the gap in evidence about help-seeking exists in relation to the specific issue of child neglect. In sum, there is little robust evidence about how parents directly signal their need for, or seek help. One of the biggest limitations is that most studies take cases of substantiated neglect as their starting point – thus information about the earlier stages is less available.

However, there are some interesting pointers from studies that approach the issue from a different direction. For example, there is some information about the potential for parents to signal the need for help that can be drawn from a study of maternal self-report. Two hundred and forty-six mothers of new-born babies in the US completed a measure of parenting concerns while still in hospital: 1.4 per cent identified specific concerns that they might neglect; 8.2 per cent worried that the father might neglect and 25.7 per cent were concerned that they might not provide good enough care (Combs-Orme, Cain and Wilson 2004). Mothers' concerns at birth were significantly related to levels of stress measured on a Parenting Stress Index 6 to 12 months later. Higher levels of stress measured on this index are associated with elevated scores on The Child Abuse Potential Inventory (CAPI) (Milner 1986). The CAPI and other such checklists have flaws and cannot be used predictively (Taylor, Baldwin and Spencer 2008) and the study is based on a series of associations. However, it does suggest that mothers of new-borns may be able to articulate their anxieties if asked.

Another study showed that mothers are prepared to self-report maltreatment. In an Egyptian study 89 per cent of 210 mothers reported some form of maltreatment of their children – most likely some form of emotional or physical abuse (Atta and Youssef 1998). Only 13.8 per cent were prepared to admit to physical neglect; however, 43.8 per cent reported neglect of safety, 53.3 per cent neglect of medical care and 46.1 per cent neglect of education. The authors themselves suggest that the findings of this study were highly culturally bound:

> …the proportion of mothers who indicated neglecting their children's needs was lower than those who reported subjecting them to abusive treatment. This might be attributed to the characteristics of families with Middle Eastern roots where mothers tend to put aside their individual interests and attend fully to their children needs. (p.4)

This highlights the influence of the wider social context on what people may, or may not, be prepared to discuss and relates to the issues of stigma as discussed later. Cultural variations in constructions of what might be stigmatizing should always be considered. Increasingly practitioners are likely to encounter parents and children from a wide range of cultural backgrounds – many of whom have moved from a different country of origin. Therefore, the study also provides a useful reminder of the need to expect that shame and stigma may be attached to a range of different concerns and may affect the issues that parents are, or are not, prepared to discuss with practitioners.

These studies raise the intriguing question as to whether people are prepared to say more to researchers than to representatives of formal systems. Researchers are not in a position to offer much in the way of ongoing support, but they do offer a level of anonymity that may free people to discuss their concerns. As many jurisdictions move towards a greater emphasis upon the need to share information between disciplines, there is a greater danger of driving people away from *all* services. The concept of 'shared responsibility' (HM Government 2010) has the potential to be interpreted by vulnerable parents as shared responsibility to separate them from their children. Cooper has suggested the need for a 'space for negotiation' that would allow for some confidentiality to enable parents to seek help without the fear of being catapulted into an investigative protection system (Cooper, Hetherington and Katz 2003).

On the other hand people do often say that it would have been helpful if someone had just asked the right questions. The block could as equally be due to reluctance on the part of professionals to 'open a can of worms' and hear things that they may have to act upon. Most researchers will now include information about the limits of confidentiality in their consent procedures which means that the willingness of people to talk about sensitive subjects cannot be attributed only to anonymity and confidentiality. Perhaps something can be learned from research methodology about ways to engage with people. In qualitative research, especially, considerable time and thought is given to the development of the interview schedules. In keeping with many practice models, interviews tend to begin with open questions and reserve prompts and more closed questions for occasions when respondents are more reticent. Practitioners who undertake research in their own agencies can often be surprised by the amount of additional information they can glean from service users with whom they have also previously had a practice relationship. It is also an intriguing possibility that some researchers in sensitive subjects are provided with more support and back-up to cope with the difficult information they may hear than some practitioners.

In summary, there is scope for practitioners to consider whether they are prepared to ask the right questions and whether they are prepared to hear the answers. Health visitors, in particular, with the right approach, could offer the opportunity for parents to talk about their own anxieties. The majority of parents do want to offer their children the best care that they can. Very few people set out to deliberately neglect their children. Many may be willing to share their concerns under supportive circumstances.

Factors affecting fathers

These studies do not, of course, tell us anything about fathers' concerns, about which there remains a huge gap of evidence. In a small study of fathers' involvement in family centres in Northern Ireland, men reported that they would choose not to attend, but if they did they would prefer to talk to a male social worker. They found it hard to accept the problems in parenting identified by practitioners, and saw centres as being places for women and mothers (Ewart 2003).

McGuigan and Pratt (2001) undertook a longitudinal study in the US following 2544 families who were part of a programme to support at-risk families and found that families were twice as likely to have child neglect confirmed in the first five years where there was domestic abuse in the household. Domestic abuse as committed by men is, therefore, a known backdrop to neglect – but little research is undertaken that would provide evidence to help practitioners understand the role of men in neglect. The search for literature confirmed the absence of research about the factors that might be affecting the parenting of fathers of neglected children.

One study that did specifically consider the role of fathers, showed that sustained father involvement and sense of efficacy as a parent was associated with lower risk of neglect (Dubowitz *et al.* 2000). However, much more information is needed about what factors impede a man's sense of efficacy as a father and how this can be identified and assessed in practice. A study looking specifically at supervisory neglect also considered the role of men (Coohey and Zhang 2006). As noted in Chapter 1, supervisory neglect can lead to fatal consequences and Coohey and Zhang describe supervisory neglect as failure in one of three ways:

- to watch the child sufficiently closely
- to provide adequate substitute child care
- to protect from a known abuser.

The study aimed to examine how either the absence or presence of men could contribute to supervisory neglect. From analysis of 157 cases of substantiated supervisory neglect they concluded that:

> …the mother's partner plays a critical role in whether the supervision problem will continue to occur. Families in which the mother's partner was not the father of all of the children in

the home or had a drug, alcohol or mental health challenge, and in which no one understands that there is a problem with how the children are being supervised or takes responsibility for it are more likely to have a persistent or chronic problem with supervision. (p.31)

These studies raise questions about the extent to which practitioners discuss parenting with fathers. Practitioners may well discuss their concerns about the capacity of the mother with fathers and father figures – they may well also discuss the extent to which the father is able and willing to provide support to the mother. But given the evidence that professional constructs of parenting are still highly gendered, there is likely to be considerably more scope for practitioners to talk to men about their own capacity to nurture their children and to grasp what is needed to keep them safe. Of the men who are in receipt of services for substance misuse, mental health problems or criminal behaviour, many will be fathers. Therefore, practitioners in these adult services, especially services where male workers and male service users are in the majority, should incorporate overt and specific attention to issues of parenting in their assessments. Fathers who do not live with their children may also welcome the opportunity to share concerns about their children if they have fears that they are being neglected. Practitioners should bear in mind that this could be a difficult topic to broach if the men feel as if they should be doing more for their children themselves and know that they are letting their children down. Nonetheless, work with fathers is likely to be enhanced if their parenting role is explored. Opportunities to notice children who many need more help will also be increased.

Family factors

While studies on factors relating to men are rare, even rarer is the study of the family environment associated with neglect. Box 2.1 highlights one of the few studies of its kind in which observation of neglectful households showed them to be less organized, more chaotic, less verbally expressive and to show less positive and more negative affect (Gaudin *et al.* 1996).

Box 2.1 Research highlight

Gaudin, J.M., Polansky, N.A., Kilpatrick, A.C. and Shilton, P. (1996) 'Family functioning in neglectful families.' *Child Abuse and Neglect, 20,* 4, 363–377.

The aim of this study, undertaken in Georgia, US, was to examine the structures and processes in neglectful families with a view to developing guidance for remedial intervention. The study also aimed to explore the roles that males play, and the impact of substance misuse on family functioning and parenting.

The study involved 102 families where moderate neglect had been substantiated and 103 comparison families matched for demographics. Data was drawn from case records, and practitioner ratings of child well-being, parental personality traits and family function. Parents and children over 12 were interviewed in their own home and administered standardized scales. Each family was also videotaped undertaking three short tasks as a family:

- to plan an outing or activity
- to select a frequently faced problem and find a solution
- to make something with a construction toy.

The results showed that caseworkers saw families where there was neglect as 'less healthy; less able to resolve conflicts; less cohesive; dramatically less well led; and less verbally expressive' (p.367). The mothers, themselves, reported more 'unresolved family conflict, and less open expression of positive feelings' (p.367). Also:

> By their own report adult males in both groups of families played minimal roles in child rearing or support for the mothers. Only four indicated that they provided any emotional or tangible support. Only half indicated occasional casual play with the children. (p.367)

In relation to the observation there was considerable variation between and across neglect and comparison groups – but on average the analysis of the videotapes indicated neglectful families to exhibit:

> less shared family leadership; less closeness, and less clear internal family boundaries; poorer negotiating skills; more vagueness in verbal expression; less willingness to assume responsibility for their actions; less responsiveness to other family members statements; less warmth; more unresolved conflict; and less empathy towards one another. (p.368–369)

The authors suggest that assessment for intervention should take account of the uniqueness of each family but should focus on what emerged to be the critical dimensions of how 'power and leadership is exercised, how well-organized the family is' and 'family cohesion/ closeness', 'clarity of internal psychological boundaries' and 'expression of positive and negative feelings' (p.371). The authors also provide detailed tables of suggested interventions depending on the nature of the problem.

Where families appear to be chaotic and leaderless, lacking in structure and boundaries, poor at problem-solving and less expressive of feelings, intervention suggestions include:

- structural family therapy
- reinforcement of adult roles
- anger management
- teaching problem-solving skills
- help with identifying and expressing feelings
- help with responding to children
- teaching positive communication
- reinforcing strengths.

Where leadership is more dominant or autocratic, and families are isolated, and show disengaged, vague or inconsistent expression of feelings and empathy and little expression of warmth, intervention suggestions include:

- teaching more democratic child management skills
- teaching parents to play with children
- teaching non-aggressive conflict resolution
- teaching problem-solving
- help with identifying and expressing feelings
- encouraging expression of positive feelings
- teaching empathic skills.

Where leadership is already democratic and egalitarian, intervention should focus on reinforcing good examples of communication, boundaries, problem-solving and conflict resolution.

The authors acknowledge the limitations of the study, especially the use of standards of 'good family functioning' that may not be culturally universal; nonetheless they suggest that careful analysis and observation of family functioning can help with tailoring appropriate interventions.

As well as providing useful evidence on family functioning, the methodology used in Gaudin *et al.*'s (1996) study may offer a helpful practice suggestion to assist with assessment. Part of their study entailed videotaping the family undertaking a few short tasks and then analysing the interactions. Practitioners could well incorporate such methods into their assessments of families where neglect is alleged. Not only could it be helpful to analyse the nature of family interactions, families themselves could also be involved in watching recordings of their interactions and reflecting upon their family functioning.

Substance misuse

Substance abuse is also known to be the backdrop to many neglectful situations. The research appears to agree that households where one or both parents or carers are drug dependent are likely to be more unstable with chaotic environments and that children may be exposed to drug-related activities. Others have discussed the association of drug misuse with sexual behaviour, including unwanted pregnancies (Cash and Wilke 2003), lower or unpredictable forms of supervision leaving children unattended or exposed, more punitive forms of discipline and perhaps more disagreement between partners on disciplining children.

An interview study in the UK with 30 recovering heroin addicts who were parents showed that people could very effectively articulate the impact of their substance misuse upon parenting (McKeganey *et al.* 2002). Parents described the extent to which they had 'not been there' for their children and could painfully articulate distressing levels of emotional and physical neglect:

> 'As much as I thought and believed I was a mother before, I wasn't, do you know what I mean? It's myself I was thinking about all of the time...' (p.236)

In many cases, available money and household resources were used to sustain the adult's drug use rather than to buy food and clothes:

> '...And it was one night, when I'd sold all the furniture in the house and the children were really starving and, instead of running about trying to get them food, I was running about trying to get my drugs. In the end I think the shame caught up with me, and the guilt.' (p.237)

Parents identified disrupted routines such as meal times, bed times, and getting to and coming home from school, mood swings of parents, and elder siblings in the family taking on quasi-parental roles for younger siblings. Parents were concerned about the knowledge that children had gained about the use of drugs and associated behaviours such as drug dealing and stealing.

This study was undertaken once the parents were well on the way to recovery, and as the authors state, it might be much more difficult for parents to acknowledge these issues at a stage when they are still in the throes of addiction. While acknowledging that these parents were committed to recovery, the study shows very clearly that, when asked, people have the potential to reflect upon their parenting capacity. It suggests that, at some level, parents who misuse drugs are aware of the impact upon their children – they may attempt to minimize the effects and are likely to resist hearing messages from concerned friends and family, but they can often experience underlying guilt. Indeed, it is possible that guilt and anxiety about the effects of the addiction upon the children could, ironically, fuel ongoing drug use in attempts to block out those feelings. The findings suggest that those who work with people who misuse drugs must take account of the parenting role – not only will this increase the likelihood that children will be helped, it will enhance practice with these adults for whom being a parent is a vital part of their life.

Interactions between factors

Factors such as parental substance misuse and poverty are well-established to be associated with referrals and registrations for neglect. The behavioural signs of their presence can be seen as indirect signals that more help may be required if children are to be cared for appropriately. However, no factor can be seen as an absolute predictor because of the number of children experiencing such circumstances who are not neglected. A number of studies in our review aimed to identify the characteristics and interactions that distinguish between children who will be neglected and those who will not. It would be very helpful for practice if it were possible to pick out the situations where neglect is most likely to occur. However, it is difficult to draw overarching conclusions from these studies, because they have different starting points and measure different constellations of factors, but there are some useful pointers for identifying who may need additional help.

On a population-wide basis Gillham *et al.* (1998) found significant correlations between rates of male unemployment and rates of registration for neglect (although correlations were higher for physical abuse). A number of US-based studies have aimed to find the factors that distinguish between those in poverty who neglect their children and those who do not.

The extent to which their findings are generalizable to the UK is unclear. Scannapeico and Connell-Carrick (2003) compared two groups in similar levels of poverty – 94 where there was substantiated neglect and 154 where there was not – and found maltreatment to be elevated in circumstances where there was an impoverished home environment, fewer parental resources and a previous history of maltreatment. Children in poor families who were judged to be more vulnerable, fragile and unprotected were more likely to be identified as maltreated than those who lived in better resourced households.

Similarly Ondersma (2002) compared 101 families where neglect was substantiated and 102 families where it was not, but there was involvement with child welfare agencies. In the context of poverty the aim was to compare the relative predictive ability of substance misuse, depression, low social support and negative life events for neglect. Negative life events were related to neglect, but the strongest predictor was substance misuse. The rate of substantiated maltreatment, most of which was neglect, was two or three times greater in infants who were prenatally exposed to illicit drugs.

Focusing more closely, Carter and Myers (2007) started from substantiated neglect cases with the aim of refining predictive models. From the analysis of 431 neglect cases they confirmed the correlation with poverty, but also found that caregivers were twice as likely to have physical neglect substantiated if they had mental health or substance misuse problems.

Wright and Birks (2000a) argue that the role of poverty in neglect and abuse has been over-emphasized in the past. Other stressors, such as poorer health and increased stress levels, could be at play. Poverty may indirectly cause greater stress, poorer health and result in early child bearing (Carter and Myers 2007). A number of studies agree that home conditions such as poor sanitation, overcrowding, and larger numbers of children in the home are significant (Carter and Myers 2007; Connell-Carrick and Scannapieco 2006; Scannapieco and Connell-Carrick 2005). Some argue that parents in poverty may shield their children to some extent by prioritizing limited resources towards the needs of their children (Burke *et al.* 1998; Edwards 1995). Families who neglect their children may live in more dangerous and less well-serviced communities where there is a lack of services and, difficulty in accessing adequate health care (Carter and Myers 2007; Thyen *et al.* 1997).

Rather than starting from cases of substantiated neglect, Cash and Wilke (2003) took parental substance misuse as their starting point with the aim of delineating the factors that would distinguish between people who neglect their children and those who do not. They undertook a secondary analysis of data from a longitudinal study in the US of men and women in a community-based drug and alcohol treatment programme. A sub-sample of 1404 women with children under 18 was identified and evidence collected within an ecological model focusing on the mother's history, current risks to herself and family, and community risk factors. With the backdrop of substance misuse the study identified factors that heightened the risk of neglect. Significant maternal historical factors included:

- the experience of sexual abuse in childhood
- having had an alcoholic parent
- history of substance misuse in the extended family.

Current risk factors included:

- use of cocaine or heroin by parent
- severity of drug use
- anxiety
- being African American.

Community factors that increased the risk were:

- having a high risk substance misusing network
- being in receipt of public assistance
- having difficulties finding childcare.

However, the likelihood of neglect was reduced when mothers:

- perceived themselves to be fair parents
- had higher levels of family interaction.

The authors note that the study is limited because of the lack of comparative data from a community sample and the use of self-report. However, the findings help to identify the factors that, in association with substance misuse, contribute to the risk of neglect.

These findings are complemented by those of Nair *et al.* (1997) who found in a study of 152 women who misused substances that those who were least likely to provide ongoing primary care for their babies in the first 18 months were:

- younger
- heroin users
- had two or more children

- had other children in foster care
- and reported depressive symptoms.

In a later study, Nair *et al.* (2003) also demonstrated the impact of the sheer number of risk factors. They examined the impact of 10 risk factors on the parenting of 161 women known to be misusing substances. They measured:

- maternal depression
- domestic violence
- non-domestic violence
- family size
- incarceration
- no significant other in home
- negative life events
- psychiatric problems
- homelessness
- severity of drug use.

Women experiencing more than five risk factors reported greater parental stress and potential for neglect. The effect of such accumulation was also demonstrated in a longitudinal study that followed 644 US families from 1979 to 1993 and analysed the risk factors for officially recorded and self-reported child abuse and neglect (Brown *et al.* 1998). Poverty, large family size, maternal sociopathy and maternal youth were key risk factors associated with neglect. Where no risk factors were identified, maltreatment and neglect was reported in 2 per cent of cases, but this increased to 15 per cent where four or more risk factors were present.

Overall, and whatever the starting point, the evidence from these methodologically rigorous studies offers strong evidence for the need to view constellations of adverse factors as indirect signals of the potential need for help. The overwhelming effect of poverty is a strong feature, as is the corrosive power of an accumulation of adverse factors. The case study in Box 2.2 illustrates how many factors can come into play and how many children may be affected.

Box 2.2 Case study Sarah

Sarah is a 34-year-old mother of 6 children. Her eldest child Jayne is 16 and is White Welsh. Jayne lives with and has been brought up by the maternal grandparents in a town 20 miles from Sarah. Sarah has a turbulent relationship with Jayne. Sarah's other children are also White Welsh. Peter is 13 and his natural brother Martin is 10. Peter and Martin's father is currently serving a prison sentence for drugs-related offences. Peter and Martin live with their mother, step father Justin, and three half siblings Jason aged five, Keith aged four and Rachel aged two. All children are physically healthy. Sarah and Justin both suffer from depression, Sarah has had a recent diagnosis of schizophrenia and Justin is alcohol dependant. The family live in a three bedroom house, on a deprived housing estate in the South Wales Valleys. Sarah and Justin are in receipt of state benefits.

All children living in the property have witnessed domestic abuse by Sarah's previous partner and now Justin. Social services were contacted by teachers at Martin and Jason's school as the boys were coming to school unkempt, not in uniform, without breakfast and on their own. Teachers had observed the brothers having 'near misses with cars' when crossing the road. Due to Justin drinking at night and Sarah adjusting to her medication, morning routines were very poor/non-existent. The children were left to their own devices to get up and go to school. Poor routines in the evenings were adding to this problem as the children were not getting to bed until late and were often woken up by their parents arguing and/or the police attending the property. The younger children were not enrolled in nursery or school and were not waking up in the mornings until 10am.

Due to the seriousness of the incidents that were reported to the social services, it was decided that an initial child protection conference would take place. During the child protection conference it was unanimously decided that the children living at the property would have their names added to the child protection register under the categories of neglect and emotional abuse. A core group was held shortly after the conference where Sarah, Justin and all agencies working with the family would meet to discuss and agree a child protection plan. The family were allocated a social worker and the social worker chaired the meeting.

At the core group Justin's alcohol support worker advised the group that Justin had attended all appointments with him and that

Justin was continuing to reduce the amount of alcohol that he was drinking. Justin's support worker also told the group that Justin had been visiting his GP regularly to have his anti-depressant medication monitored. Justin then spoke and expressed his feelings about how this positive change had impacted on the routines in the home. The social worker chairing the meeting recommended that Justin continue regular meetings with the alcohol support worker. Sarah's community psychiatric nurse then spoke and confirmed that Sarah's medication has been significantly reduced due to potential risks as Sarah is now pregnant. Sarah and Justin commented on this and told the group that Sarah is managing well with the reduction. Teachers from the schools then took their turns to speak to the group and advise of the absences and lateness that the children's class teachers had recorded in their register. The teachers both agreed that although there are still incidents of absence and lateness these have become fewer and the children have been appropriately dressed and clean. The support worker from a voluntary support organization informed the core group that the family have been available for all planned contact with the Family Outreach and Support Service and have engaged positively. The worker explained the work that was being carried out regarding routines and boundary setting. The family's allocated social worker spoke and recommended that Sarah attend the local Freedom Programme which is a course for women that have been affected by domestic abuse. The allocated social worker then summarized the meeting and confirmed all actions of the family and the agencies involved.

Help-seeking

The studies referred to in the previous section did not explore whether parents would be prepared to seek help as a result of their concerns or actual behaviour and there is little exploration of help-seeking. There is limited evidence to help understand whether parents whose children are neglected try and fail to seek help, or whether they tend not to seek help from professionals. The evidence suggests that it should not be assumed that parents or children will seek help in response to experiencing the factors associated with neglect. The issue was touched on briefly in a small study in the UK (Appleton and Cowley 2004). The primary focus of the study was on the role of health visitors in identifying families in need – but the authors comment:

the…assumption that clients in need will contact the service is negated by data from the client interviews, which reveals how difficult it can be for vulnerable people to seek out professional help. (p.794)

The paper includes a quote from a mother:

'And, say, next week, if I had a problem, I'd find it hard to ring up about it…because you don't like to be a nuisance…' (p.792)

This is congruent with other evidence. Mothers of neglected children tend to have low self-efficacy, to have little belief in their own ability to change and that others can offer anything to help (Crittenden 1996). They may have learning difficulties and may have had experiences of the system that did not feel supportive. Mothers and fathers of children who are referred for neglect are increasingly likely to be misusing substances (Home Office 2003) and may be reluctant to seek help for fear of losing their children.

Ghate and Hazel (2002) found an association between the use of informal and formal help, some parents accessed both, some neither. As part of the evaluation of Sure Start people who had not used services were interviewed about the blocks to access and expressed many of these views:

…parents with extreme problems such as drug or alcohol related abuse, mental health problems, domestic violence or criminal records were reluctant to be drawn into 'systems'. They were frightened. They did not want to be on anyone's list. They had learned not to trust professionals… A long timescale is needed to break down such barriers and to establish relationships with families with this level of resistance. (Anning *et al.* 2007, pp.81–82)

This was similar to the views of parents interviewed in a study of child protection, parental substance misuse and domestic abuse. The parents were aware of the impact of their circumstances upon their children but were afraid to be honest about their problems in case their children would be removed (Cleaver *et al.* 2006). This issue is highlighted in the UK government's policy response to an analysis of families at risk – *Think Family* (Cabinet Office 2007b):

Most families with multiple problems are likely to have had considerable experience of mainstream services, such as the child's school or the family's GP, as well as contact with specialist services. However, their engagement with services may often have been chaotic and it requires a level of coordination beyond the capacity of the individual frontline worker or indeed that of the clients themselves. (p.26)

The Children's Plan (DCSF 2007a) responds to the issue by pledging an expansion in good-quality outreach associated with Sure Start Children's Centres. The problem has also been identified in Scottish policy documents:

Often parents, children and young people do not seek help from services because they think that this would label them as either bad or neglectful parents or as an offender. They do not want to face intrusive investigations or enquiries which do not actually lead to any help for them. (Scottish Executive 2005, p.10)

Broadhurst (2003) points out that much of the literature to date on help-seeking is based on inferences rather than empirical research. Research tends to have been undertaken with those who have been referred for services, which is clearly limited because it misses information about people who may need some support but do not come to the attention of services. In the light of the prevalence statistics described in Chapter 1 it is safe to assume that many children experiencing neglect commensurate with those known to services do not come to the attention of those in a position to help. Broadhurst reports on her review of health and welfare literature on help-seeking in relation to what she describes as 'stigmatizing problems'. The aim is to provide evidence to help with understanding the processes in force before referral to, or accessing services, with a particular emphasis on understanding the person as an *active* agent rather than merely a passive recipient of intervention. She summarizes what are known as 'early stage models' of help-seeking that identify three stages:

1. Problem definition.

2. Decision to seek help.

3. Actively seeking help. (p.342)

The reviewed literature suggests a divergence between the ways in which problems are defined by professionals and how they are defined by the target user group. The literature tends to focus more on the former than the latter – thus we have more information about how needs may be constructed by professionals and organizations than by parents themselves. She cites a study about mothers with children with Attention Deficit Hyperactivity Disorder (Arcia and Fernandez 1998) that provides a very interesting reversal of the predominant discourse about access to support:

> *Mothers* are referred to as 'the gate-keeper' to services, indicating that it is how mothers define problems which determines how, when and why they will ask for help. (p.344)

She points out that much of the evidence about the psychological aspects of help-seeking in relation to family support derives from the study of people already involved with services, and particularly child protection processes. Drawing on the broader literature some emergent themes emerge, including concepts of ambivalence, loss of control and fear and stigma and a form of 'cost-benefit' analysis of the consequences of seeking help.

One rare study did consider the circumstances associated with families who had approached the social services in England for help (Tunstill and Aldgate 2000). Interviews were undertaken with the main carer and some children at the time of referral and six months later. It was found that:

- Many families had been struggling for a long time with a high level of need before approaching social services.

- Those who were professionally referred had more chance of getting a service than those who approached Social Services themselves.

- A third of the families received no services. The most requested form of help, social work support, was least likely to be met.

- The benefits anticipated and obtained by families were stress relief, help with child development, improved family relationships and alleviation of practical problems.

- The main needs expressed by children were for support, help with schooling and resolution of family conflict. (p.236)

So, this study shows that even if people do come and ask for help they may not get it, or may not get the kind of help they want or need.

Practitioners who work on the cusp between formal and informal support, and professionals in universal services, are in a potentially highly influential position in that they can act either as positive ambassadors for the formal system or frighten people away from taking further steps into the helping system. A recent review of the literature on early intervention and prevention also identifies this issue:

> Effective intervention with children depends not only on the *fact* of involving their parents, and sometimes wider family, but also on the *way* of doing so. The examples in this publication repeatedly demonstrate the importance of engaging parents in a collaborative approach, building on their strengths and taking

account of their views and experiences. They highlight the need to recognise the problems that families themselves often face and to develop strategies that build confidence and capacity to enable parents to properly fulfil the crucial role they play. They illustrate the vital part that outreach work often plays in making contact with families who would otherwise miss out on services, but who can often be successfully drawn into both universal or specialist (targeted) provision. (C4EO 2009, pp.7–8)

The review provides helpful examples of services which have built in effective engagement processes.

Policy documents are scattered with references to parents as 'hard to reach'. *Think Family* gives a brief comment on the ways in which parents might find access difficult. However, our review of the evidence suggested that there is far more scope for services to carry out an analysis of the extent to which they may be 'hard to access'. The labels 'hard to reach' and 'hard to change' are extensively used and appear with little or no definition in many policy and research documents (Cabinet Office 2007b; Faugier and Sargeant 1997; Kandel 1975; Thoburn 2009). What are the implications of holding up a mirror to the helping system? Would parents and children describe help as being easy to access and easy to use? The evidence from the research studies reviewed would suggest that people do not find services very easy to access or engage with (see also Box 2.3). And the repetitive nature of serious case enquiry findings would certainly suggest that our systems are hard to change.

Box 2.3 Activity

Are services easy to reach and easy to use?
Consider the following vignettes and think about the many factors that can get in the way of seeking help and what can be done to smooth access to support.

1. Tom, who is worried about the care his young child is receiving from his ex-partner, would like to speak to someone to get a bit of advice about what to do. After some searching in an old phone book at his mother's house he finds a number for social services. When he rings the number on his pay-as-you-go mobile an automated voice tells him that the number to call has been changed and gives him a different number. He calls that number

---

which is a general switchboard for all council services and which has an automated routing system. After selecting social services he holds for around 20 minutes before someone answers. He is only able to briefly mention his concern before he is asked to hold again at which point his phone credit runs out.

2. A local voluntary family support service has left lots of colourful leaflets in the community encouraging people to come and see what is on offer at their family centre. Sally is desperate for some babysitting so she can get a break, but she feels there is no one that she can ask to look after her baby who cries a lot and her toddler whom she describes as 'hyperactive'. She goes to the centre where, Jo, a very friendly staff member greets her and gives her a cup of tea. When Sally describes what she needs, Jo explains, very regretfully, that they ask that parents and children come to the centre together where they can take part in lots of joint activities. He finds a leaflet about a local babysitting circle but Sally realizes that this means she'd have to offer to babysit other people's children in return which really scares her. She leaves disappointed.

3. Sara and Jim's child, James, has physical and intellectual disabilities. Sara is starting to find it hard to physically lift James and attend to his care, and Jim works long hours to try to make enough money to cover their mortgage. Sara hears that there is a local self-help group for parents with disabled children. She goes to a meeting but finds that the group is currently preoccupied with a campaign to prevent the closure of a school for disabled children. She finds the anger and outrage of the other parents alienating because she can't understand why people would want their children to be in specialist rather than mainstream provision. She has never seen herself as political and is scared that if she is labelled as a trouble-maker she and Jim won't get any more services from the council.

4. Since a young age June has used drink and drugs to relax. She now has three children and is aware that she is becoming more and more reliant on drugs and alcohol just to get through the day rather than for fun. She knows she is spending too much on substances and is getting really frightened about her level of addiction. So far she believes that she has managed to mask her dependence from her partner, friends and family. After weeks of working up to

seeking help she takes a bus to the city centre where she knows there is a counselling and support service – as she approaches the service she sees a near neighbour of hers leaving the building. She immediately hides in a shop door and gets the next bus home.

5. Kevin is thirteen and has experienced three spells in foster care with three different sets of carers, as a result of physical and emotional neglect. To date he has had four different social workers and has attended three different schools where he has encountered more teachers than he can remember. He has been to many review meetings which have been chaired by many different people. He has been registered at three different GP practices and has never seen the same doctor on more than one occasion. Kevin has lots of worries about his parents, about his siblings, about himself. He knows he is very behind in class and that he can't read properly which is embarrassing – but there is no one that he knows well enough to talk to.

Overall, the research suggests that we still have much to learn about what would support parents to come forward and ask for help. Figure 2.1 illustrates some of the many ways in which the need for help can be directly or indirectly signalled. Practitioners from all settings should be alert to all these possibilities.

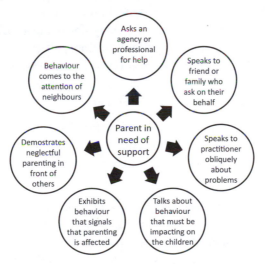

Figure 2.1: Showing some of the many ways in which a parent may signal a need for more support with parenting

Implications for noticing possible neglect

The findings from studies like those discussed above can yield what seem like a baffling array of factors without providing practitioners with clear messages to help with recognizing whether more support is required. The evidence about parental characteristics associated with neglect is very complex and few clear-cut pathways have been identified. Nonetheless, there is still an urge to try to pin down what may be predictive factors. For example, the UK *Action Plan on Social Exclusion* (Cabinet Office 2007a) asserts that the government

> will develop and promote better prediction tools for use by front-line practitioners, for example health visitors and community midwives, and will seek to ensure that those identified as at risk are followed up. (p.9)

The evidence from the studies we analysed suggests that such tools cannot discriminate sufficiently and that the emphasis should be more upon assessment of need. Concerns have previously been raised about the accuracy of screening instruments to identify children who will be abused or neglected (Taylor *et al.* 2008). The problem lies not so much with the tools themselves, but the dangers inherent in relying on the predictive powers of such tools. No tools can guarantee against false positives or false negatives and therefore practitioners will always need the skills and knowledge to make sound professional judgements, even if they make use of tools to assist with their assessments. Brandon *et al.* (2008) also suggest that assessment tools cannot take the place of good professional judgement. However, they indicate that while risk assessment tools may not improve risk prediction, tools to assist with the analysis of information collected in assessments may be helpful. Their findings in relation to serious case reviews should encourage practitioners to look beyond presenting problems when families are in crises. As Aldgate and Rose (2008) state:

> Practitioners wanting a fail-safe checklist, in whichever discipline they are working, will fail to find one and practitioner judgement will always need to play a part in identifying and responding to risk. (p.12)

So – although the studies may not help with developing a fail-safe predictive model, they do confirm practice wisdom about the effects of these factors upon parenting, and suggest that it is the accumulation of factors that may especially erode parenting capacity. As Cleaver *et al.* (2006) found in their study in England:

...domestic violence or parental substance misuse rarely exist in isolation. Many families experienced a combination of domestic violence, parental alcohol misuse, drug misuse, mental illness and learning disability. When domestic violence and parental drug or alcohol misuse coexisted the effect on all aspects of children's lives was more serious. (p.5)

Practitioners who encounter adults who appear to be, or are open that they are, affected by factors such as substance misuse, domestic violence or mental health problems should ask themselves if there is likely to be an effect on parenting. They should also be prepared to ask the parents themselves about their perception of the effects on their children. It is especially important for practitioners to be alert to situations where parents are facing an accumulation of stressors. This may become apparent to health visitors, for example, if parents describe some of the factors they are facing. Schools may also become aware of the number of pressures that are affecting parents if they are having a knock-on effect on children's attendance, demeanour and performance. Practitioners working in adult support services will be in a very good position to see the range of factors that may be interacting to erode parental capacity. Any practitioner who has contact within the family home may also be able to observe, and respond to, the direct effects in the domestic arena. In summary, in keeping with the theme of Chapter 1, in many ways recognizing neglect is not that complicated – it requires practitioners to ask themselves and ask the person if what they are experiencing is reasonably likely to affect their parenting.

KEY MESSAGES

1. There needs to be greater attention to the position of parents who need help but are not accessing services.

2. In relation to people already known to services it is helpful to understand their journey to support.

3. The evidence supports practice wisdom about the associations between neglect and parental factors such as substance misuse, mental health problems and domestic abuse. These factors usually occur against a prevailing backdrop of poverty.

4. Practitioners from all professions should be proactive in seeking creative and supportive ways to ask people about their parenting concerns, and consider some of the lessons from research methods.

5. The preponderance of research into maternal circumstances must be complemented by more research on the paternal experience.

6. Assessment should focus on the accumulation of stressors and incorporate an historical element.

7. Policy should prioritize the support of good assessment skills rather than the development of predictive 'tools'.

8. Policy initiatives aimed to improve engagement with 'hard to reach' parents should be complemented by strategies to ensure that services are not hard to access.

9. Further research is needed into the conditions that support parents to seek help when there is a potential for neglect.

10. All practitioners need to remain alert to the direct and indirect signs that parents need more support and therefore that their children may be experiencing some form of neglect.

3

Signs that Children's Needs are not Being Met

Introduction

As we suggested in Chapter 1, the preoccupation with trying to decide whether the label 'neglect' should be applied to a child's experience can deflect from focusing on the child's unmet needs. We argue that the sharper and narrower definition should be reserved for situations where it is required to underpin compulsory measures. For other situations we suggest that a wider definition based on unmet need is more helpful. For example, the disparity between prevalence and incidence figures suggests that there are many children and parents who would benefit from more support on a voluntary basis and where wider definitions would be helpful. Of course, some caution is needed here. It is unwise to assume that just because a child has not appeared on the radar of the statutory system their circumstances would not warrant some form of compulsory intervention. There are also occasions where very serious and entrenched neglect can be engaged with on a non-compulsory basis. But the overall message is that the broader the definition, the more likely it is that children with unmet needs will be noticed and supported.

In the previous chapter we explored some of the factors that have been shown in the research to be associated with erosion of parenting capacity. Much of this research will chime with practitioner experience and wisdom. It is all too often very clear that children's lives are blighted when they are surrounded by the fall-out of problematic substance misuse, domestic abuse, parental mental health problems, lack of parental resources and support and poor domestic management skills. In this chapter we focus more closely on children's experiences of neglect and the ways in which their needs for additional help may be signalled either directly or indirectly. As with parenting, there is very little research into what would support children to seek help on their own behalf but we have included some pointers from the literature.

It may be obvious that one of the simplest ways to identify neglect would be to recognize the signs in a child's development. And neglect does certainly affect children's development. The difficulty is that neglect can affect so many different developmental domains and can affect developmental trajectories in so many different ways that there is no one obvious 'marker' of neglect. Nonetheless, any sign of compromised development should be a cause for concern and should prompt further curiosity about the reasons. If it turns out that there is another reason for the problems, then that is also very useful information if something can be done to help the child.

Although we describe some of the signs of neglect in children this does not mean to imply that one should *wait* until there are signs to act on behalf of children whose needs are not being met. The evidence about the devastating long-term effects of chronic neglect should be the spur for prompt action before a child's development is seriously compromised. The starting point is the question:

• What does this child need to grow and develop?

Signs of neglect in children

There is an existing significant body of evidence about the impact of neglect upon the emotional, behavioural, physical and cognitive development of children (Egeland, Sroufe and Erickson 1983; Gaudin 1993b; Horwath 2007; Stevenson 1998; Taylor and Daniel 2005). A child's developmental trajectory is supported by responsive caring that ensures that physical, emotional and cognitive needs are met; by the same token that trajectory will be suppressed when needs are not met. Practitioners with a basic knowledge of child development should be able to pick up signs that something is amiss with development, even if they cannot be certain of the cause.

Physical development

Common physical manifestations of neglect include stunted growth, chronic medical problems, inadequate bone and muscle growth, and lack of neurological development that negatively affects normal brain functioning and information processing (Glaser 2007). Processing problems may often make it difficult for children to understand directions, may negatively impact the child's ability to understand social relationships, or may make completion of some academic tasks difficult without assistance or intervention from others (Twardosz and Lutzker 2010). Lack of adequate medical care may result in long-term health problems or impairments such as hearing loss from untreated ear infections. Nutritional neglect occurs when a child is undernourished or is repeatedly hungry for long periods of time, and can sometimes be evidenced by poor growth. If proper nutrients are not available at critical growth periods, the child's development will not follow the normal and usual pattern (Weavers 2009). Health professionals should notice these signs in one of two ways. If children are being seen regularly then their compromised development will become evident from signs such as departure from expected growth trajectories and evidence of untreated conditions (such as dental caries). It is often said that neglect goes less noticed than physical abuse because of the absence of obvious signs such as bruises and broken bones. However, neglect does manifest itself viscerally – it is written in children's bodies and lack of growth is as good as evidence for action as a bruise. If children are not being seen regularly then their invisibility to the health care system can be a sign of neglect which should be followed up.

Medical neglect encompasses a parent or guardian's denial of or delay in seeking needed health care for a child. This may be manifested in different ways. There can be denial of health care, which is the failure to provide or to allow needed care as recommended by a health care professional for a physical injury, illness, medical condition, or impairment. Delay in health care is the failure to seek timely and appropriate medical care for a serious health problem that any reasonable person would have recognized as needing professional medical attention (DePanfilis 2006). Examples of a delay in health care include not getting appropriate preventive medical or dental care for a child, not obtaining care for a sick child, or not following medical recommendations. Not seeking adequate mental health care also falls under this category.

There may also be chaotic use of services. If the parental lifestyle is associated with frequent moves and difficulties with domestic organization then there may be disorganized use of services. Parents may be slow to register with a medical practice or use hospital and out-of-hours services. With this kind of service use there is a real danger that no health professional will have access to an overview of the child's pattern of physical development. It should not be understated that around a third of children who become the subject of a serious case review in England or Wales for neglect (because they have died or are seriously injured or there has been a 'near miss') have a history of missed health care appointments

(OFSTED 2010). Friedlaender's study in the US showed that seriously maltreated children were 2.62 times more likely than non-maltreated children to have had one change in primary care health provider in the previous year, and 6.87 times more likely to have had two or more changes (Friedlaender *et al.* 2005). Frequency of attendance and rates of diagnosis were, on the other hand, not significant.

Two studies conducted in specialist burns units offer a sobering perspective on ways in which neglect may be signalled physically. In the US Hultman *et al.* (1998) found the average age of a group of 21 children whose burns were related to neglect to be 2.7 years (as opposed to 2.1 for burns associated with physical abuse). Burns due to both abuse and neglect were likely to be scalds. The majority of these children had been identified to be at risk before their injuries, yet were returned to their original environments. Where children suffered neglect families often delayed seeking help (19%) and neglected children fared worse than abused children in keeping appointments and receiving adequate wound care. Chester *et al.*'s (2006) UK study focused more specifically on neglect. The cases of 440 children admitted to a burns unit were reviewed in detail by a multi-disciplinary team who identified that 4 were due to physical abuse, 21 due to neglect and the rest to accidents, thus indicating a greater prevalence of burns from neglect than abuse. They found the burns to have more in common with those related to accidents than those related to abuse and that where a child was neglected it was more likely that:

- the child had not been given first aid at the time,
- there was a delay of over 24 hours before seeking help,
- the burns would be deeper.

The authors highlight the value of having a social worker and social work assistant attached to the unit to carry out assessments and home visits and that assessment cannot be replaced by 'algorithms' for recognition.

In another hospital-based study Thyen *et al.* (1997) examined the records of 5446 children admitted to hospital in Massachusetts and Connecticut and identified concern about abuse in 2.5 per cent of the sample and neglect in 3.1 per cent. Cases admitted to hospital with concerns of physical abuse were most frequent in cases of head trauma, whereas concerns for neglect were about children who had been admitted for head trauma and also for toxic ingestion. Again there had often been delay in bringing the children to the attention of medical practitioners.

Emotional development

Secure attachment relationships develop in the context of sensitive and responsive care. They are recognized as providing the optimum environment for psychosocial development. Drawing on the work of Howe (2005) and Crittenden (1999), Stevenson (2007) summarizes the effects of different patterns of neglect upon the development of attachment. She describes 'disorganized' neglect as characterized by chaos and crisis, where parental behaviour is driven primarily by feelings. As a result of the parents' preoccupation with their own feelings and wishes babies and young children do not get the kind of responsive consistent interactions they need and so can develop demanding and fretful patterns of interaction. Where there is 'depressed, passive and physical' (p.52) neglect, characterized by withdrawn and dulled parental characteristics akin to depression and learned helplessness, the children can become very listless. These children learn very early on that there is no point in demanding attention.

Turney (2005) describes the close interconnection between the provision of physical care and the accompanying emotional investment. She challenges the assumption that mothers *should* care and 'naturally' care for children. Instead she suggests that practitioners should look at all the possible caring adults around the child, including the father. Practitioners should also recognize that the capacity to care is affected by interpersonal relationships and wider environmental factors. Therefore practitioners should assess the quality of each parent's relationship with each child and the meanings of those relationships. This may also mean accepting that some mothers may not be able to 'care' for or about their children. Practitioners should also look at the wider context and their influence upon parents and look more widely at the human resources available to the child in the wider community.

Practitioners with even a basic understanding of attachment and what secure attachment between a child and carer looks like can, at the minimum, recognize when adult–child relationships seem to be awry. The way in which parents and children relate to the practitioner can also provide hints about their template for relationships.

Cognitive development

The suppression of cognitive development is one of the most damaging effects of neglect. Children's capacity to think, make connections, understand the work of people and objects, play around with ideas and concepts – all these things are less likely to develop in the absence of a consistent adult foil for their questions and an adult spur for their curiosity. The development of language and thought are closely connected and both are stimulated within the context of secure attachment relationships. The neglect of both physical and/or emotional needs in the early years is likely to affect the foundations of cognitive development.

In the early years it is during many of the routine acts of physical care that cognitive development is stimulated. Sometimes assessment frameworks and written reports fail to capture just how fundamental very simple everyday interactions are. It may sound rather clinical but things like playing peek-a-boo while pulling on a child's top helps them with object constancy; showing that a full cup spills while an empty one does not helps with understanding liquids. With older children things like naming colours and counting are instinctively stimulated by parents and carers during getting dressed or eating breakfast and so on. When out shopping attentive parents point things out to their children – they name objects, ask children to say what sound a dog makes or a cat makes, they point out basic connections like 'it's sunny so it's warm', or 'there's clouds in the sky so it may rain'. And if children have early contact with other children who are a bit older than them, and other interested adults, the scope for stimulation is vast. People, including people who are also practitioners, know these things. So when they see a child who is left for hours in a cot; a child who is strapped for hours in a buggy in a corner of a room; a child whose questions are never answered, they should know that cognitive development and the associated emotional intelligence skills are not being nurtured.

Cumulative harm can be illustrated here. Children with suppressed cognitive skills, who have had little opportunity to feel what it feels like to think about something and have that thinking supported will undoubtedly struggle when they start school. They are the children who have the most to gain from consistent and regular attendance. And yet they are the children who are most likely to have erratic attendance. They are the children who need to be the most alert and attentive, and yet they are the most likely to be tired, hungry and listless. Many of the early problems with learning can be attributed to neglected children's poor language development (Stevenson 2007). A study comparing the effects of different forms of maltreatment found:

> The neglected children demonstrated a decline in functioning during the early school years. They were significantly lower on all achievement subtests, and by second grade all of the neglected children were referred for special education services. In general, these children had difficulty coping with the demands of school. (Egeland 1991)

A study in the US found that both physically abused and neglected children showed greater social and behavioural problems at school as judged by teachers – neglected children showed more externalizing problems and the greatest academic delay (Depaul and Arruabarrena 1995). The fact that these research findings were based upon teacher ratings demonstrates that the signs were evident and suggests that teacher ratings can be as useful to practice as to research.

Disadvantages accumulate: as these children get older their behaviour may become more challenging – partly because they are very behind in class and are therefore upset, anxious, embarrassed or really have got beyond caring; partly because they are not receiving consistent and appropriate boundaries for behaviour at home. As they get older, for many neglected children their challenging and difficult behaviour is the block that prevents them from receiving sympathetic, kind and nurturing responses from the adults they encounter. Instead they hear a barrage of exhortations to 'behave' – but many of these children do not really know what 'behaving' feels like.

Cumulative harm is also a helpful concept when considering the needs of neglected teenagers. Stein and colleagues undertook a literature review (Stein *et al.* 2009) and developed materials for young people and for practitioners focusing specifically on issues for teenagers (Hicks and Stein 2010). In some cases it is during teenage years that neglect is first experienced, often as a result of changes in family composition. But for many young people it is during teenage years that the accumulation of the effects of years of neglect can be felt very keenly and be manifested in a number of ways. In teenage years neglect may not be associated only with omission of care because some acts of commission may occur such as abandonment, being forced to leave home, or becoming included in drug cultures. They note that it is important to 'look at *patterns of neglect over time* and recognize the impact of both acute and chronic neglect' (Hicks and Stein 2010, p.9). They suggest that young people themselves often under-estimate neglect, they may have become used to their parents' behaviour and have a loyalty to their families, 'Young people might think it is their fault that they're being neglected, so they go along with it (young person's view). Tables 3.1 and 3.2 are taken from the multiagency guide for practitioners and show some of the causes and some of the consequences of teenage neglect. The messages for practice are helpful and act as a reminder to look beyond immediate presenting issues. Many young people who are considered to be 'troublesome' will have a background of neglect.

Table 3.1 Thinking about: Causes of adolescent neglect, reproduced from Hicks and Stein (2010) p.13

Research Review	Issues for practitioners
Disabled young people	Experience higher rates of neglect
	Communication impairments may make it difficult to tell others what is happening
	Being isolated, not receiving regular services may increase likelihood of neglect
	Practitioners need to distinguish between what is a result of disability and what are signs of neglect
Looked after young people	Many experience neglect before being looked after
	This may include neglect of their physical health, education and emotional needs
	Importance of promoting stability and secure attachments through high quality of care
Impact of parental problems	Mental health problems, substance and alcohol misuse increase likelihood of neglect
	These problems often increase parents' emotional unavailability
	Young people more likely to be left alone, lack parental supervision and positive role modelling
Young carers	Being a young carer may increase the likelihood of neglect
	Parental problems may also mean older children and adolescents may be drawn into caring, to the detriment of their own care
	Young people may not receive support at key developmental stages, such as puberty, early and later adolescence
	Lack of supervision and boundaries may result in young people being exposed to greater likelihood of harm and experiencing more problems

Table 3.2 Thinking about: the consequences of neglect and the *Every Child Matters* outcomes reproduced from Hicks and Stein (2010) p.14

Every Child Matters	Issues for practitioners
Being healthy *Physical health*	A quarter of serious case reviews were carried out on 11 to 18 year olds – many of these included a history of childhood neglect
	Ensuring young people have appropriate medical attention
	Recognizing the importance of adequate food and diet
Mental health and well-being	Recognizing anxiety, depression, low self-esteem and proneness to suicide
Risky health behaviours	Drug and alcohol abuse and early sexual activity
Staying safe	Close association between parental neglect and young people running away from home; substance misuse; sexual exploitation and risky sexual behaviours; and potentially young people being stigmatized and bullied by their peers
Enjoy and achieve	Neglectful parenting associated with poor academic achievement and misconduct at school
Make a positive contribution	Neglectful parenting associated with anti-social behaviour, young people getting into trouble; and violent conduct
Achieve economic well-being	Experience of neglect, and consequences identified above, can be cumulative and contribute to poor outcomes in adulthood, including education, employment and well-being

Types of neglect and impact

Longitudinal Studies of Child Abuse and Neglect (LONGSCAN) is a consortium of research studies in the United States. The consortium operates under shared by-laws and procedures. The coordinating centres are based at the University of North Carolina, with satellite sites at Baltimore, Chicago, North Carolina, San Diego and Seattle. Each site is undertaking a separate study on the aetiology and impact of child maltreatment.

As part of the LONGSCAN studies, Dubowitz and colleagues broke down neglect into sub-types:

- physical neglect
- psychological neglect
- environmental neglect – defined by risks in the neighbourhood
- cumulative neglect – defined by a combination of the other sub-types.

In a series of studies they examined whether there were links between different sub-types and outcomes of children at different ages. They also explored whether sub-types had better predictive power than the general category of 'neglect' as used by child protective services (CPS) and looked at different conceptualizations of neglect. The studies were prospective, detailed and complex and just a few key findings are summarized here:

- psychological neglect was associated with increased levels of internalizing and externalizing behaviour in children at age three (Dubowitz *et al.* 2002)

- caregiver failure to provide for basic needs and verbally aggressive behaviour towards a child was associated with delays in language and communication, socio-emotional adjustment and behavioural problems at age four (English *et al.* 2005)

- psychological neglect was associated with teacher report of problems in peer relationships and externalizing behaviour at age six (Dubowitz, Pitts and Black 2004)

- environmental neglect was associated with parental report of increased internalizing and externalizing behaviour in children at age six (Dubowitz *et al.* 2004)

- general neglect as identified by CPS was associated with behaviour problems, impaired socialization and problems with daily living skills at age eight as was the specific neglect of medical needs (Dubowitz *et al.* 2005)

- with a sample of socio-economically deprived children the sub-types identified different children to be experiencing some form of neglect at six than had been identified by the CPS, suggesting the sub-types picked up a wider range of neglectful circumstances (Dubowitz *et al.* 2004). However,

- with a sample of children already subject to CPS referrals there were moderate correlations between the sub-types and neglect as identified by CPS; and the associations with child outcomes at age eight were similar (Dubowitz *et al.* 2005).

The findings are not clear-cut and could not be used predicatively without large numbers of false positives and negatives. Overall, though, the studies point to the importance of considering compromised development and behavioural problems as potentially indicative of neglect. Trying to associate one particular kind of neglect with one particular set of outcomes may not be terribly helpful: '…interest in disentangling the types of neglect represents a form of misplaced precision, given the complexity of children's lives' (Dubowitz *et al.* 2005, p.508).

Neglect associated with domestic violence, parental substance misuse and parental mental health problems

The association between neglect and each of domestic violence, parental substance misuse and parental mental health problems alone or combined is clear (Cleaver, Unell and Aldgate 1999; Kroll and Taylor 2001). These factors often co-exist with other structural disadvantages that in themselves are associated with neglect such as poverty, poor housing and lack of resources. As suggested in Chapter 2, practitioners who become aware that any or all of these may be a feature in a child's life should be alert to the potential for neglect. While it is very likely that children will be affected by these parental factors, not all of them will necessarily also experience chronic neglect, although they may experience other forms of trauma and disruption. In some cases they may experience some fluctuations in capacity and intermittent neglect without the rest of their development being seriously compromised. But in many situations these parental factors are associated with a wider neglect of children's emotional and physical needs. If this is the case, then the children are at risk of all the effects of neglect described earlier. The key message for practitioners is to be alert to the signs that children may need some additional support, whether they fit the official criteria for 'neglect' or not.

Excessive drinking or drug-taking and smoking during pregnancy can affect the developing foetus (Cleaver *et al.* 1999). Babies can be born with physical addictions to substances. Many parents whose children are neglected also neglect their own care, thus women may not eat well during pregnancy or make use of health services. Physical violence by men towards women during pregnancy can also pose a risk to the foetus and indeed some men may direct their violence towards the unborn child. Therefore, practitioners who work with pregnant women and their partners are in a position to pick up early signs that the care and protection of the growing foetus is being neglected. Pregnancy can provide a window of opportunity for change, but it can also be a time of anxiety, defensiveness and vulnerability. Sensitive practitioners can find ways to connect with a parent's hopes for their baby and the knock-on hope for change in their own lives. If parents experience empathic, but appropriately challenging support during pregnancy they are likely to be more open to ongoing support with parenting. Clumsy, judgemental or confrontational approaches may, on the other hand, drive people away from services and expose the baby to greater risk of undetected neglect. It is also unhelpful if practitioners show no interest or concern about potential damage to the foetus or young baby because, in effect, this acts as tacit acceptance of the harmful activity. It can also send strong signals to the parent that their unborn child does not matter, which may mirror very much how they feel about themselves.

Children's perspectives have been aptly captured by Gorin (2004) in a review of studies of children's experiences of domestic violence and parental substance misuse and mental health problems. They summarize some of the effects on children that have been identified by Cleaver *et al.* (1999) which include

> feelings of fear, sadness, anger, anxiety, guilt, concern for their parents, low self-esteem; bed wetting, sleep and eating problems, aggressive behaviour, withdrawal, running away; problems at school or in developing peer relationships; social isolation; inappropriate caring responsibilities for their age. (Gorin 2004, p.7)

Each of these characteristics could develop as a result of other forms of trauma; children who have experienced the loss of a parent, for example, might exhibit bed wetting or problems at school. Essentially, if children are distressed by home circumstances they are likely to show some signs, either by internalizing or externalizing behaviour. Teachers and other professionals should be in a position to recognize childhood distress and should be interested in finding out whether some help is needed. Often appropriate help can be provided without the need for invocation of formal child protection proceedings.

Based on a number of different studies Gorin (2004) indicates that the likelihood of poor outcomes is exacerbated if children have to provide extensive care to parents and if their education is disrupted. When parents are absent from home acquiring drugs or drinking or undertaking criminal activity then there is a risk of physical neglect and absence of adequate supervision. Neglect of physical and emotional needs is also associated with taking drugs or drinking or the after-effects. Times of withdrawal can be difficult for children because parents may be anxiously preoccupied with obtaining a further supply, may feel unwell and may be emotionally absent. Children whose parents misuse drugs may also be at elevated risk from sexual abuse as a result of exposure to dangerous people and lack of adequate supervision. When children's need to be kept safe is not met, then 'neglect' leads to dangers of 'abuse'. This is just one example of the extent to which neglect and abuse can be intertwined.

Some of the children living with parents affected by these factors may have received adequate or good cognitive stimulation, albeit sometimes on a fluctuating basis. Some will have not. As Gorin found, formal education is often affected by erratic attendance and poor performance when at school. There may be frequent changes of school due to chaotic lifestyles. It can be especially difficult for mothers and children who are trying to hide from a violent man because they may be found via schools.

The emotional impact of these factors can also be profound, especially as children are often aware that something is not right at a young age and younger than parents realize. Erratic and frightening behaviour by parents can affect their emotional development and sense of security. Some of this is illustrated by a quote from a child:

> 'Mummy likes to drink a lot and it doesn't mix with her medicine and her medicine doesn't mix with the, what she drinks and she'll forget what she's doing when she drinks and she like starts talking a lot and the next minute you know she's like speaking into another world and that's what gets me really confused when I don't understand what she's talking about. She'll start asking funny questions. She'll be sleeping on the floor, weeing and going to the toilet in the wrong place.'
> (Aldridge and Becker 2003 cited in Gorin 2004, p.15)

Of course, in relation to recognition there is often a considerable amount of secrecy and taboo. Secrecy within the home can be damaging enough for children, but the secrecy may be especially salient outside the home. Many of these children and their parents would be terrified at the prospect of 'the authorities' becoming involved. To be fair to teachers and other practitioners children can be very good at covering up what is happening at home. But there are a range of possible routes by which a child in need might be noticed including extended family, members of the community, other children and their parents, health professionals, housing officials and adult services.

Another way by which children's need for support could be signalled is if it becomes apparent that they are undertaking significant levels of care for parents. This is, again, not a straightforward area. There are many strands to the debate about young carers. Gorin found that in the studies they reviewed in many cases the process of children helping out at home was managed reasonably and children were involved in negotiations about what they did or did not help with. Situations can, on the other hand, veer into emotionally neglectful if there is no additional support and children feel there is no choice but to assist.

Children who undertake care for parents in Wales were interviewed for a study by Thomas *et al.* (2003). The children were recruited for the study by various means and should by no means be regarded as a sample of 'neglected' children. Nonetheless, their observations are helpful. One finding came from the difficulty in locating children for the study. Attempts to recruit participants via schools and other agencies highlighted just how invisible these children can be and there was a very low awareness among agencies of these children. Many of the children interviewed valued their education and were very keen to attend and work hard, but they did struggle to attend regularly and keep up with the work, and they did not always find teachers to be sympathetic.

For young carers the impact can be physical, educational, emotional or on later adult life. The authors challenge the concept of 'parentification' and 'role reversal' because although the children talked of feeling responsibility for their parent, the majority of the children did not equate their caring with 'parenting'. In other words, the children were clear that their parent was the parent but they needed help with some aspects of their care. This is an important finding, because it is simple to slip into jargon such as 'parentified' but if this is not a meaningful concept for children it may not reflect the reality of their experience. What this suggests is that practitioners need to hear the children's perspectives rather than make assumptions. Box 3.1 provides a case study that illustrates some of these issues.

Box 3.1 Case study Naomi

Naomi (14) is a single child of White, British origin. She attends mainstream school and has no disabilities or impairments. Naomi's mother, Emma, died suddenly four years ago. Since her mother's death, Naomi has resided in the care of her father, Tom. Tom is 63 years of age. He is of White, British origin. He has been diagnosed with cancer. He is a drinker and has problems with his alcohol use which he does not always accept. The family live in a two-bedroom, privately rented, terraced house in a deprived area of an ex-industrialized northern town. Tom is in receipt of state benefits.

Naomi's school contacted the local authority children's services to report concerns about Naomi's appearance, presentation and school attendance. When social workers visited Naomi and Tom at their home the following concerns were identified:

- Unsafe, unhygienic, hazardous home conditions, for example, used tampons on the floor; faeces and urine on the floor of the toilet, mouldy food left on plates and rotting food packaging strewn around; rubbish, clutter and debris piled up everywhere. Tom said that he had not been upstairs for 12 months and that he slept downstairs on the sofa.

- Naomi's bedroom was extremely cluttered to the point that she could not get into her bed. She reported that she slept in her father's bed because it 'made her feel closer to her mother'.

- Naomi's presentation and personal hygiene were of concern. Naomi appeared grubby and dirty. She had few items of clothing that fitted her and no clean underwear. School uniform was dirty, old and unkempt.

- No soap, toothbrush, toothpaste or shampoo were evident and there were no cleaning products.

- Few boundaries, inadequate supervision and no routines were being implemented.

- Naomi had been 'speaking' to an 18-year-old male on *Facebook* and had invited him to come and stay at her home.

- Naomi would spend much of her leisure time in the pub with her father.

- Naomi had poor school attendance and low achievement.

The social worker sought Naomi and Tom's permission to refer them to a voluntary organization's neglect project that provides intensive family support. The family support workers met with the social worker, Naomi and Tom and openly shared the concerns about the neglectful care which Naomi was receiving. All agreed what needed to change and the support that the project could offer. Intensive family support was provided to the family through two to three planned and unplanned visits per week to the family home to address the issues of concern. The intervention lasted seven months.

Support included:

- Assisting, advising and guiding Tom in the development of organizational strategies such as daily planners, calendars, shopping lists and routines.

- Enabling and encouraging Tom to take responsibility for improving and maintaining the household conditions – breaking tasks down into small manageable, prioritized targets and developing maintenance routines.

- Monitoring, challenging and providing daily prompts to encourage and support change.

- Close and regular liaison with other agencies particularly children's social care, education, health and voluntary sector providers.

At the last Child in Need meeting, positive changes were identified by all including:

- Improvement in household conditions.

- Naomi's bedroom was significantly improved, Tom had purchased wallpaper to decorate it. She slept in her own bed.

- Cleaning products, toothpaste and toothbrushes, toilet rolls, towels and ample food were available.

- Naomi's appearance improved.

- School attendance and punctuality significantly improved. Naomi was in a better frame of mind to learn and was working more towards her capacity.

- Naomi completed the Seasons for Growth programme (in relation to the death of her mother).

- Tom was assessed by adult services, independent living team. Adaptations were made to encourage his independence.

- Naomi received ongoing one-to-one support though a local children's centre and took the opportunity for voluntary, part-time work in an area of her choice (hairdressing).

Child characteristics

The question as to whether there are child characteristics associated with the likelihood of being neglected has not been the subject of extensive exploration. In our literature review some hints as to causal characteristics emerged. For example, a study in the US found an association between a 'difficult' child temperament and emotional neglect (Harrington *et al.* 1998).

A study in the UK looked specifically at the issues of non-organic failure to thrive (also known as weight faltering and part of the Children Act 1989 definition of neglect) (Wright and Birks 2000b). Data on growth patterns, feeding history, parental perceptions of child behaviour and temperament was collected by health visitors at the 6–8 week check and again between 9 to 18 months in relation to 97 children identified as failing to thrive and 28 control children. Overall, the children identified as failing to thrive were positively described by their parents and, compared with the control group, were seen as shy and undemanding, had presented early problems with the introduction of solids and were described as children who liked food but significantly less so than the control group of children. The authors raise the question as to whether the children themselves have inherently less demanding personalities, low appetite and a lack of interest in food resulting in low intake and late weaning.

The issue of whether there are child characteristics associated with neglect, though, is a difficult one to explore because of the connotations of 'victim-blaming'. Smith and Fong (2004) suggest that it is very difficult to distinguish whether some child characteristics contribute to the neglect or result from earlier neglect. For example, a baby whose needs for attention have been neglected may develop into a toddler who is unresponsive to the parent. This unresponsiveness may contribute to further neglect, but is also a result of earlier neglect. They do note that children born prematurely or of low birth weight are at elevated risk of neglect, perhaps as a result of attachment disruption because of extended hospital care for the child.

It is known that disabled children are at elevated risk of all forms of maltreatment including neglect (Sullivan and Knutson 2000). Kennedy and Wonnacott (2005) draw on the social model of disability to highlight the social and structural barriers that can impact negatively upon parents and undermine the care they can provide. By the same token they also note the danger that practitioners accept lower standards of parenting for disabled children, or attribute developmental delays purely to the disability rather than consider the possibility of neglect. They provide very helpful guidance for practitioners on how to assess and intervene to support neglected disabled children.

Horwath (2007) summarizes those at greater risk of neglect as:

- children born to mothers who use drugs during pregnancy
- low birth weight babies
- children with disabilities
- the child perceived to be difficult to parent. (p.62)

The associations between child characteristics and neglect are so complex that it would never be safe, nor indeed ethical, to predict that a particular child might be neglected because of who they are. Nonetheless, it is sensible to be alert to the elevated risks for children who are born prematurely; of low birth weight or disabled. Whether a child is perceived to be difficult to parent can be very idiosyncratic and related to extrinsic factors such as being born during a time of particular stress, resembling someone who is disliked or where temperaments do not mesh. Overall, the message for practitioners remains the same; if something seems amiss with the parent–child relationship then it is sensible to try and find out more.

Help-seeking

In our literature review we found very little evidence about neglected children's direct help-seeking. From a study of calls to ChildLine (Scotland), Vincent and Daniel (2004) found that very few children would call to seek help about neglect, whereas they would call about physical abuse and sexual abuse. Carpenter *et al.* (1997) showed that the drawings of maltreated children are significantly different from non-maltreated children. The differences were not sufficiently distinctive to provide a 'diagnosis' of neglect but the findings suggest that drawings could be included as part of the assessment of possible neglect.

Hints about child help-seeking behaviour emerge in the Paavilainen, Astedt-Kurki and Paunouen (2000) study on the role of school nurses:

> According to school nurses, children tended to protect their parents and did not talk about their family affairs easily. The first sign pointing to problems was often the fact that the child consulted the school nurse more frequently than before. Young children often spoke more openly than older ones, but there were great individual differences. It was easier to make young children talk by questioning them. (p.5)

In one of the few studies of children's self-report, Kantor *et al.* (2004) describe the development and testing of a child self-report scale for neglect. The questionnaire is designed to capture the child's experience of actual behaviours relating to the meeting of physical, emotional, supervision and cognitive needs; and separately to measure the child's perception of whether their caregiver is neglectful. The questionnaire is child-friendly and is administered on a computer using pictures and choices on a scale of 'very like me/not like me'. Tested on 144 children, already identified as neglected, and 87 comparison children the questionnaire reliably distinguished between the groups. More details about a study to validate this measure can be found in Box 3.2. Using the same questionnaire Hines, Kantor and Holt (2006) found correlations between siblings' self-report of neglect, especially for more serious neglect. As with adults, these studies suggest that when using the right tools children can, and will, report behaviours related to neglect.

Box 3.2 Research highlight

Kantor, G. K. *et al.* (2004) 'Development and preliminary psychometric properties of the Multidimensional Neglectful Behavior Scale-Child Report.' *Child Maltreatment, 9*, 4, 409–428.

The paper describes the development of the 'Multidimensional Neglectful Behavior Scale-Child Report (MNBS-CR). The authors note that the majority of instruments to measure neglect rely on professional ratings and that they are often limited in their scope. The MNBS-CR was designed to both focus on the child's perspective and also to capture broad conceptualizations of neglect by incorporating a wide range of parenting behaviours. In this way the measure is not focused narrowly on 'neglect' as responded to by state systems, but neglect in a wider sense. The definition used to provide the framework for the measure is:

> Neglect is a behavior by a caregiver that constitutes a failure to act in ways that are presumed by the culture of a society to be necessary to meet the developmental needs of a child and which are the responsibility of a caregiver to provide. (p.411)

The measure was designed on the basis that items should reflect behaviors – specifically behaviors of omission and not be confounded by causes, motives or effects. The measure covers four domains:

1. Physical needs.
2. Emotional needs.
3. Supervision needs.
4. Cognitive needs.

The measure also aimed to separate children's experience of parental behaviours from their judgements as to whether the behaviour is neglectful. This is because children experiencing lack of care will not automatically describe themselves as neglected.

The measure was developed to be administered by computer using pictures with graphics that match the age and gender of the respondent and using touch-screen responses. For each question two pictures are presented on the screen, one representing a nurturing parent behaviour and another the opposite (neglectful behaviour). The child is asked to touch the picture that is most like them. A second screen then asks for a rating of the behaviour by asking whether the picture is 'a little like you; sort of like you; a lot like you; really a lot like you'. Half way through there is an interactive game to minimize boredom. Scales were developed for two age groups – 6 to 9 and 10 to 15 and after piloting with 47 children were refined to include a total of 52 items:

- 33 assessing emotional, cognitive, supervisory and physical neglect
- 7 assessing neglect linked with parental substance misuse, exposure to conflict, violence in the family and abandonment
- 6 assessing children's own appraisals of neglect
- 6 measuring depression (in the child).

An example of a physical care item is 'This girl's mother makes sure she takes a bath' versus 'This girl's mother does not make sure she takes a bath' (p.415). And an example of self-appraisal of neglect would be 'This child feels like no one takes care of him' (p.414).

The measure was then administered to 255 maltreated children, 144 of whom had been neglected and to a comparison group of 87 children in the community. There was a lot of variability in the extent to which the items were able to discriminate between the groups and the authors note the need for some modifications and further testing. However, the potential of the measure for screening and assessment was indicated by the finding that 'younger and older children with a documented history of neglect scored significantly higher on the MNBS-CR than community children' (p.424). This is, of course a group effect and it could not be assumed that it would necessarily distinguish neglected children on an individual basis. The computer-based method of administration appears to be very successful and the measure is innovative as a way of obtaining children's perspectives. One finding stands out:

> The most poignant and telling item of [the general appraisal] scale is the item indicating that the child did not feel that someone loved him or her. As anticipated, neglected children reported this more often than community children. (p.423)

There is broader research into children's views about help-seeking that can offer further insights about how to support neglected children. Hallett, Murray and Punch (2003) gathered the views of two samples of children aged 13–14 living in Scotland. One group comprised 22 boys and 33 girls in mainstream schools and the other 16 boys and 15 girls in residential units. The young people were interviewed in groups and individually, and were also asked to put notes in a 'secret box' about any worries they had that they had not shared with anyone. The young people reported worrying about schoolwork, death or ill health, parental conflict and falling out with friends. There were clear gender differences in that girls reported more worrying than boys and the difference was even more marked for young people in residential care. A common response was to tell someone, usually best friends, parents and especially mothers. Girls were more likely to tell someone than boys. However, a third reported that they would not tell anyone. Other forms of coping included listening to music; boys might hit something or pretend that everything was fine; while girls might write in a diary.

Friends were very important sources of support, especially for girls. When asked about helping agencies the young people living at home thought they would use helplines or a guidance teacher, but were reluctant to use formal agencies. They were very unclear about how one would access services and felt that GPs would be too busy to listen. Teachers and school nurses were seen to be unavailable:

> 'Sometimes she's [school nurse] really hard to find. Like at lunch time and like you cannae find her. At lunch, at breaks you don't, you can't see her. And if you're like ill in class, sometimes she's like away photocopying or away somewhere else and you can't find her.' (p.132)

Confidentiality and trust were especially important for young people. They feared that if they told adults they would take over control and do things against their will. The views of both groups were broadly similar, the main difference being that the young people in residential settings would make use of keyworkers and had a wider range of coping mechanisms, some more extreme.

The young people in Hallett *et al.*'s study were not necessarily representative of neglected children as such, but many of the messages are similar to those found in other studies. Gorin (2004) reviewed the general literature about children's help-seeking as well as in relation to the specific issues of parental substance misuse, domestic violence and parental mental health problems. One important reminder is that children do not use operational descriptions like 'domestic violence' or 'substance misuse' so immediately there may be a gap between service labels and children's perceptions of their own needs. A further extrapolation from this is that they are probably extremely unlikely to refer to themselves as experiencing 'neglect'.

Gorin (2004) describes four types of coping strategies employed by children. Each of these could potentially be evident to an alert and interested adult:

- *Avoidance/distraction* – physical and/or emotional avoidance; distraction by music or television, etc. Child may not be overtly seeking help, but excessive avoidant behaviour may be evident, especially to teachers.

- *Protection/inaction* – keeping watch on parents and on money, etc; sometimes not taking action out of fear of consequences, also may be hard to spot, but may be evident if the child is anxious about the parent while at school or at other activities.

- *Confrontation, intervention and self-destruction* – attempts to stop violence or stop parents using drugs – given that these may be fairly futile it is likely that children will have a low sense of self-efficacy in time.

- *Help-seeking and action* – not a common strategy but can include, in domestic abuse, for example, phoning the police.

The research reviewed by Gorin suggests that many children do not feel able to talk to anyone for reasons including fear of an abuser, fear of the consequences (especially if there are illegal activities), fear of being removed from their parents, or that they will not be believed. Girls are more likely to tell someone than boys, and may confide in friends. Sources of informal support include parents (especially mothers), friends, siblings, extended family and pets. Seeking formal help was unlikely to be the first recourse, apart from confidential helplines:

> They lack trust in professionals, are concerned about confidentiality and fear intervention in the family and associated loss of control over the consequences of telling. (p.59)

Children express confusion about professional roles, and uncertainty about who to approach and how to go about contacting someone, coupled with a concern about stigma.

They had mixed experiences of talking to teachers and often felt they did not help them, or felt that teachers thought their accounts were 'stories' or 'excuses'.

Listening is described as 'active' in that there are ways in which adults can actively convey their willingness to listen to a child. Children appreciate adults who look at them and try to help them. They want help and someone to assume some responsibility, but not to remove all their control. All too often adult responses appear not to be helpful: 'Adults were reported as exacerbating problems by over-reacting, causing embarrassment, taking over, moralising and/or trivialising matters' (p.53).

Similar messages emerged in Thomas *et al.*'s study of young carers (2003) in that they rarely had someone in school they could talk to. Their views of social services were largely negative but they were very positive about young carers' projects, especially because they met their need for someone to talk to.

A consultation event about the English child protection system yielded very rich information from children and young people aged 10 to 18 who had contact with various agencies (CRAE 2003). In relation to neglect specifically the young people had many suggestions about how neglect could be manifested including:

'Like where the mum and dad are not being a mum and dad to their children. They're just letting children do what they want... They're not making sure children are fed and watered [and] not making rational decisions – like my mother.'

'They might be acting like the parent and not having time to look after yourself.'

'You mightn't be getting what you need at home, for example, food, privacy, pocket money, showers and toiletries.'

'They might smell dirty – no one would like to sit near them.'

'If they're tired and falling asleep in class.'

'Teachers need to pick up on learning difficulties and let children and young people know what sort of help is available out there.'

'Notice whether parents come to pick children up from school. If didn't come there's something wrong – go and see if child is alright. Keep a close eye on them.' (pp.9–10)

These are strikingly similar to the 'signs and symptoms' commonly included in training courses for professionals.

The main factors in seeking help were knowing and being able to trust someone, especially someone who cared about the young person, including family members (especially mothers), but also some practitioners. Confidentiality again emerged as a big issue:

> 'If you told a teacher they wouldn't keep it safe, they'd tell other teachers.' (p.11)

They did not want things to 'spiral out of control', they wanted to be able to trust someone and be able to talk over their concerns; but equally they wanted people to provide help. Much of the findings are congruent with work undertaken in Scotland to develop a Children's Charter – for more details see Box 3.3.

Box 3.3 Activity

In Scotland a 'Children's Charter' was developed by Save the Children on behalf of the then Scottish Executive (Scottish Executive 2004 #6664) as part of a child protection reform programme. It was based on extensive consultation with children and young people and was shaped by their views on what they wanted from professionals that they may encounter. As stated in the Charter:

This is a message to all of us – politicians, communities, parents, families, neighbours; as well as police, health, social work, and education authorities; and people who work directly with children and young people – about what is important to them and how we go about helping to protect them. (p.1)

Devised to cover all forms of maltreatment, it is highly congruent with the evidence from research studies about how children prefer to be helped. It is also eminently transferable to other jurisdictions and can be applied specifically to children who may be experiencing some form of neglect.

1. Look at the Charter and consider each of the messages about what children expect of professionals who may be in a position to help them.

2. Consider the extent to which your agency respects these wishes.

3. Consider the extent to which your individual practice with children meets these expectations.

4. Are there aspects of policy and practice that could be adjusted to better meet these requests from children?

> ### The Children's Charter
> Get to know us
> Speak with us
> Listen to us
> Take us seriously
> Involve us
> Respect our privacy
> Be responsible to us
> Think about our lives as a whole
> Think carefully about how you use information about us
> Put us in touch with the right people
> Use your power to help
> Make things happen when they should
> Help us be safe

Children talk a lot about the importance of friends, but there is very little information on how peers can be supported to deal with concerns about neglect. And yet, as shown in a recent survey of 3000 8–12 year olds many children are aware of, and worry about their neglected peers:

- almost two thirds (61%) had seen suspected signs of neglect this year
- on average children saw at least three children with some of the signs of neglect this year
- more than one in ten (13%) told us they'd seen suspected neglect nine times this year
- children as young as eight are seeing signs of neglect in their peers. (Action for Children 2010, p.3)

Signs included children not having friends, wearing ill-fitting or smelly clothes; being unwashed or dirty; not getting meals; being bullied, laughed at, ignored or talked about. If children are aware of these signs there is no reason why teachers should not be also.

Overall, the research on children's help-seeking shows how incongruent their needs are with an investigative-driven system and one that requires all practitioners to 'report' or 'refer' concerns as soon as possible. While it is clear that children want adults to provide actual help, they do not want precipitate action that removes all their control and which breaches their confidentiality and trust. Clearly it may not be possible to provide a system that is both totally confidential and effective in protecting children from serious harm. But it is clear that flexibility and sensitivity are required if children are to feel safe talking about their worries.

Implications for noticing possible neglect

What emerges from the research is that the signs of neglect should be apparent at quite early stages to practitioners in a range of settings. Indeed, there can be signs before birth and then during infancy. The evidence suggests that children may show behavioural signs of neglect by the age of three. Psychological neglect is shown to be particularly damaging. Again, though, the evidence suggests that it is not possible to pinpoint very specific links between neglectful parenting and particular effects on children. Despite the lack of specificity, the evidence about the cumulative harm associated with neglect is compelling and it confirms the value of early intervention, an issue that is discussed in more detail in Chapter 6.

Children themselves can give very articulate accounts of the neglect they see in their peers. Teachers and other professionals can provide very good evidence for research studies. It is highly likely that there are many practitioners who are worried about many children because they are observing the physical, behavioural and cognitive manifestations of neglect. So it may not be that people are not noticing neglect, rather that they are not very sure about what to do next. In the next chapter we will explore the barriers to action, some of which are exacerbated by the nature of the kind of systems to be found in the UK and other jurisdictions with similar approaches.

The evidence about children's views gives a mixed picture about what would help. But perhaps what they need is best summed up by Aldgate and Statham (2001):

> In the end, what children want is straightforward: enough food, warmth, adults who love and nurture them, consistency, achievements and to be treated with dignity as befits their status as child citizens. (p.95)

KEY MESSAGES

1. A broad definition of neglect based upon the concept of unmet need and closely related to understandings of child development is most helpful for children.

2. Any signs of delayed development in any domain should arouse the curiosity and concern of practitioners.

3. The physical impact of both emotional and physical neglect can be manifested at an early age, with some effects on development beginning before birth. Effects on physical and mental health can be wide-ranging and lead to permanent disabilities.

4. Multi-disciplinary teams in hospitals, including social workers and social work assistants, can assess the likelihood of a burn being associated with neglect.

5. All children need the secure base of at least one secure attachment relationship, but neglect is highly associated with insecure attachments.

6. The nature and meaning of all relationships between all the adults in the family and the child should be assessed. The impact of the adult relationships and the wider context should also be considered.

7. Cognitive development can be seriously impaired by neglect and the cumulative harm can be manifested in serious problems in school and during adolescence.

8. When practitioners become aware that parents may be affected by substance misuse, domestic violence or poor mental health then they should immediately consider the likelihood of effects upon the children.

9. Some factors can elevate vulnerability to neglect including pre-birth exposure to drugs, low birth weight, disability and having characteristics that render the child 'hard to parent' by their own parent/s.

10. Children prefer to seek help from family and friends and are unlikely to turn to formal help as a first port of call. They are more likely to speak to adults who appear to care about them and who will listen without taking precipitate action.

4

Responding to Children whose Needs are not Being Met

Introduction

Having covered the evidence about the ways in which children and parents may directly or indirectly signal their needs for help, in this chapter we consider the evidence about whether and how these signs are noticed and acted upon and some issues to bear in mind when undertaking assessments. Neglect is complex and can raise nagging worries for people – they may know something is not quite right, but are not sure how not right something needs to be before they do anything. And then once they have decided they need to do something (and all sorts of things can get in the way of making that decision), they are unclear about what the exact something might be. This is possibly especially so for lay people – the concerned neighbour or bus driver – but we know that professionals struggle as well. Teachers for example might have intuitive worries about a particular child, but faced with a lack of evidence, clarity and confidence about what to do, may hesitate about taking action.

Recognition and response tend to be lumped together in policy and research, and in many ways there is considerable overlap between the two – for example, fears about dealing with the child protection system may affect the extent to which someone is open to noticing signs of neglect. And noticing a child in need and choosing not to do anything is still a response. As we will discuss later, the term response can also cover a range of different phenomena. It tends to be associated with 'reporting' or 'referral' but from the child's point of view response includes everything about the way in which the adult responds and relates to them and their circumstance either directly or indirectly.

Recognition

From the evidence provided in Chapters 2 and 3 it should be clear that, in many cases, there will be ample indications that a child and his or her family may need additional help to prevent neglect. And yet, many children remain in need to the extent that their development is seriously compromised.

General public

It is instructive to return to the studies of Rose and her colleagues described in Chapter 1 (Rose and Meezan 1995, 1996; Rose and Selwyn 2000). They found that members of the general public tended to give vignettes depicting abuse and neglect higher ratings of concern than professionals. The studies were not designed to explore the reasons for such differences, and nor do they provide evidence about developmental outcomes, but they do suggest that the general population is at least as well equipped as professionals to *recognize* aspects of neglectful care, if not more so. And yet, professionals are also members of the public and it seems paradoxical to think that professional training and experience would render someone less able to recognize signs of neglect. There must be other factors at play.

Rose and Selwyn (2000) argue that understandings of neglect within the UK are influenced by:

- the role of the definer
- the current political and economic climate with narrower definitions of neglect during times of scarce resources
- the time period when a definition occurs, i.e. parenting behaviour may remain constant, but what is considered the norm may change
- the legal framework supporting a definition
- the societal context within which the definition is framed.

Dubowitz *et al.* (1998) also suggest that different professionals from different disciplines may employ different definitions reflecting their background, training and the purpose of the definition. An example would be the findings of a Scottish study in which social workers rated statements about children's care which showed that social workers tended to place greater value on emotional than physical care (Daniel 1999b). As discussed earlier, the evidence also suggests that operational definitions of 'neglect' can affect the number of children receiving a service. Such variations in definition potentially contribute to differences in expectations about when a child's care should cause professional concern.

The most direct research evidence about professional recognition of neglect relates to health staff whereas studies involving education staff and police are rare and studies of social workers tend to focus on response.

Health staff

Paavileinen *et al.* (2002) found that of 513 nurses and physicians in a children's hospital in Finland, two thirds believed that they could recognize maltreatment despite the associated difficulties. For physical abuse bruises would be obvious signs. But in answer to open-ended questions respondents identified a number of aspects of child and parent behaviour that would assist with identification. Child behaviours included fearfulness, shyness, aggressiveness, lack of trust and crying, while parent behaviours included over-protectiveness, aggression, shunning or evasiveness, haste or being under the influence of alcohol or drugs. All these are congruent with the research evidence described above. The things that made identification difficult were 'awkwardness of the phenomenon, the staff's pressure of work and relative unfamiliarity with the phenomenon' (p.287). Although neglect was not separately addressed, overall, the study suggests a reasonable level of confidence among these staff about their capacity to recognize maltreatment.

In a further study of the views of 20 experienced public health nurses in Finland, Paavilainen and Tarkka (2003) examined how they define child abuse and how they identify child abuse. The nurses divided abuse into two categories – physical and emotional. Aspects of neglect fell into both categories – physical neglect included failure to attend to needs or actions such as failing to give the child required medication, giving them alcohol or drugs to keep them quiet, leaving them alone or failing to send them to school. Emotional neglect was seen to include paying no attention to the children, failing to set them boundaries, indifference and showing no interest in their activities. Identification was supported in two ways, by 'tools' for identifying abuse and 'markers' indicating abuse. These insights about identification (recognition) are very helpful and capture some useful practice considerations. Tools include:

- *knowledge acquisition* – essentially describing a process of initial assessment involving asking further questions, gathering information from others, undertaking further health checks on the child

- *interactive skills* – describing skills of verbal and non-verbal communication with families
- *intuition* – relating to the professional experience that helps with picking up signs
- *capacity for handling problematic situations* – involving undertaking proper groundwork and perseverance.

These are illustrated by the quotes from nurses:

> 'I've learned to make more direct questions. You cannot afford to jump to conclusions. I feel I've gained more courage with the years.'

> 'It's feeling…that something isn't right. It's an instinct and a feeling of something being terribly wrong. I guess it comes from tiny details when you link one thing to another.' (p.52)

Markers for maltreatment include:

- *Child behaviour and appearance* – identifying 'cries for help' such as psychosomatic symptoms, frequent consultation with the school or public health nurse, lack of cleanliness, etc.

  > 'Parents may starve the child, and this is why the child's blood values are poor.' (p.53)

- *Family behaviour* – noticing ways in which the family may isolate itself, secrecy, avoidance, defensiveness, poor relationships and lack of social support:

  > 'They are lonely and have no social networks, grandmothers or others. They have no friends. They are so busy with their own lives that there is no time for the children. The children are left on their own.' (p.53)

Despite describing this useful combination of knowledge and skills the authors acknowledge that more work is needed to support nurses with intervention following identification.

The mention of intuition by these public health nurses is interesting, because it is a concept that tends to cause some system anxiety and yet it may be part of the constellation of human characteristics that impels people into helping professions in the first place, and, if given its place can be a helpful element in recognition (Helm 2010).

Ling and Luker (2000) discuss the way in which intuition or 'gut feeling' in the realm of the nursing profession is often rejected as unscientific. They undertook an ethnographic study of health visiting practice in England by interviewing 18 health visitors and 6 nursing officers and directly observing home visits and case conferences. Health visitors described using intuitive awareness both reactively and proactively, indeed, cases were described where health visitors had tenaciously followed up concerns they attributed to intuitive awareness. Intuition was seen as a complex process: 'intuitive awareness encapsulates empathy which is "honed by experience" together with the intellectual abilities developed because of the academic content of their training...' (p.575). The health visitors distinguished intuition from the kind of 'objective' knowledge used when writing case notes. Intuition was seen as something that could not be written about but it was seen to be important to be able to talk about it. We would argue that recognition of neglect will be enhanced if skilled practitioners are able to acknowledge their intuitive awareness and have the opportunity in supervision or case consultation to integrate knowledge based on intuition with knowledge based on theory.

Other studies provide the most direct evidence about the extent to which health visitors in the UK are equipped to recognize that children may be in need of help. Ninety-two health visitors completed a questionnaire in which they were asked to rate the importance of 45 signs and symptoms of neglect (Lewin and Herron 2007). There was considerable agreement about the five that were rated as most serious: violence to the child, the child being excluded by the family, the child being left unattended or left to care for other children, violence within the home and a domestic atmosphere of high criticism and low warmth. There was less agreement and lower ratings for factors described as those that 'might traditionally be expected to be central for health vistors', (p.102) including poor weight gain/nutrition, under-stimulation, developmental delay and untreated infestations.

The findings suggest that health visitors are equipped to recognize the importance of the parenting and emotional aspects of neglect. This is supported by the findings from a survey (n=58) and interviews (n=12) with health visitors about their work with 'vulnerable' families (Appleton 1996). The emergent concerns were not so much about recognition as about problems of identifying resources for the families. Indeed the health visitors indicated that they were able to identify a wider range of vulnerable children than would be picked up using the trust's formal criteria. In a similar vein Appleton and Cowley (2004) describe the inconsistent and patchy application of formal guidelines and assessment checklists for the identification of families in need, and question the value of such guidelines for improving outcomes for families:

> We recommend that health visitors seriously question whether it is ever appropriate to attempt to replace professional judgement by the apparent shift towards greater adoption of general and invalid formal guidelines in health visiting practice. (p.796)

Overall, these studies suggest that health visitors in the UK are well-equipped to recognize signs of neglect. There is less empirical information about the views and practice of the medical profession in recognition. The UK National Institute for Health and Clinical Excellence (NICE) guidelines on child maltreatment offer health care professionals a summary of some concrete features that should alert them to possible neglect, many of which do not require health expertise and can also be considered by other practitioners:

> Abandonment, bites (animal), clothing, dirty child, failure to thrive, faltering growth, footwear, head lice, health promotion, health reviews, home conditions, immunisation, lack of provision, lack of supervision, medication adherence, parental interaction with medical services, persistent infestations, poor hygiene, scabies, screening, smelly child, sunburn, tooth decay. (National Collaborating Centre for Women's and Children's Health 2009, p.5)

There is more detail in the guidelines which also include some very helpful and down to earth messages:

> Instances of inadequate clothing that have a suitable explanation (for example, a sudden change in the weather or slippers worn because they were closest to hand when leaving the house in a rush) would not be alerting features for possible neglect...
>
> Achieving a balance between an awareness of risk and allowing children freedom to learn by experience can be difficult. However, if parents and carers persistently fail to anticipate dangers and to take precautions to protect their children from harm it may constitute neglect...
>
> Children often become smelly or dirty during the course of the day. However, the nature of the child's smell may be so overwhelming that the possibility of persistent lack of provision or care should be taken into account. Examples include:

- ° child seen at times of the day when it is unlikely that they would have had an opportunity to become smelly or dirty (e.g., an early morning visit)

- ° if the dirtiness is ingrained...

It may be difficult to distinguish between neglect and material poverty. However, care should be taken to balance recognition of the constraints on the parents' or carers' ability to meet their child's needs for food, clothing and shelter with an appreciation of how people in similar circumstances have been able to meet those needs. (pp.12–13)

It is interesting that these guidelines about early recognition do not call upon sophisticated nursing or medical knowledge – they draw pretty much on common sense. That is not to say that medical expertise is never helpful in recognition of neglect – the research on burns described in Chapter 2 being an example.

While dentists, like any other person encountering children, may observe general signs of neglect such as a child being apparently under-nourished, they are in an especially strong position to pick up signs of dental neglect. In the US dentists have an ethical obligation to familiarize themselves with signs of abuse and neglect and to report suspected abuse or neglect and in some states dentists are additionally subject to mandatory reporting legislation. Importantly dentists in the US are not only expected to observe signs of abuse in the oral area but to consider any wider signs of abuse or neglect (Sfikas 1999).

Dental neglect may occur alone, but it is highly likely to one part of a pattern of wider neglect. Dental neglect can also have emotional consequences because of the associated discomfort. The definition used in the US and the UK is:

> wilful failure of parent or guardian to seek and follow through with treatment necessary to ensure a level of oral health essential for adequate function and freedom from pain and infection. (American Academy of Pediatric Dentistry 2003, p.13)

As Kellog highlights (2005), the associated pain and loss of function 'can adversely affect learning, communication, nutrition and other activities necessary for growth and development' (p.1566). She underlines the importance of distinguishing between parents with inadequate knowledge or access to resources, from 'wilful' failure. She clearly locates the role of discussing these issues with the dentist and suggests that referral on to child protection services should only occur after attempts have been made to provide information and practical support for access to services as well as reassurance that the child will not experience pain during treatment. The combination of empathy and authority described is sensible and helpful.

While there is not mandatory reporting in the UK the Department of Health provides helpful guidance for dentists with a clear message that:

> Safeguarding children is not just about referring them when you have concerns but is about changing the environment to ensure that risks to their welfare are minimised. (Department of Health 2006)

Education staff

The role of education professionals is picked up in some of the studies that use multi-professional subject groups or some that describe characteristics of children – however, the lack of empirical research into the views and practice of education staff is striking. The bulk of the literature on early recognition is in the form of practice guidance, protocols, lists of signs and symptoms or information on training. There is some research on factors that affect referral which is considered below, but none of these studies met the criteria for our systematic review. Many studies allude to the importance of schools and teachers; many studies allude to the severe impact of neglect upon cognitive development, but there is little empirical research on neglected children and the ways in which they engage or not with schools and education.

Social workers

The studies in our systematic review confirmed the existing evidence about the role of social workers as gatekeepers to services. They also confirmed that by the time children come into contact with social workers they have often already experienced periods of neglect. Social workers in the statutory services in England and in many countries with similar jurisdictions have become increasingly shunted towards the statutory child protection end of the support continuum. The vision of early intervention and integrated practice set out in many policy documents raises questions about the future role of social work. If early intervention and family support become increasingly the preserve of the universal services it is not inconceivable that social work could become even more of a residual service reserved for situations where there is a need for investigation and compulsion. On the other hand, it could be argued that the skills of social workers in relationship building and assessment are helpful for early recognition of signs of potential neglect as well as being helpful for early intervention and family support. In reality, though, a model of early intervention increases the number of parents and children eligible for services, thus stretching the existing resources. Either way, there needs to be clarity about the envisioned social work role and a comprehensive analysis of the required accompanying resources. Otherwise social services will continue to be pulled in both directions and will be unable to fulfil either function effectively.

Response

Research on response by the general public and professionals other than social workers tends to conceptualize response as 'referral' or 'reporting'. As shown in Figure 4.1, some evidence has accumulated about factors that affect practitioner willingness to act, that is, to report.

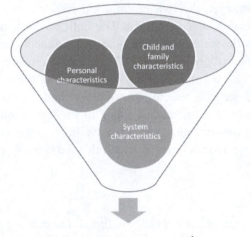

Willingness to report/act

Figure 4.1: Showing what the evidence indicates about the different influences upon practitioner willingness to act upon signs of neglect

Four studies from the US address the issue of referral systematically (Ashton 2004; Bryant and Milsom 2005; Hansen *et al.* 1997; Mitchell, Turbiville and Turnbull 1999). Although all include a range of maltreatment there was sufficient allusion to neglect for them to meet our inclusion criteria and their findings about the factors that affect response are summarized in Table 4.1.

Table 4.1: Showing evidence drawn from four studies about the factors affecting referral/action by different professionals

Ashton (2004): 276 entry level social work students
Bryant and Milsom (2005): 263 school counsellors Hansen *et al.* (1997): 125 psychologists and 85 social workers Mitchell *et al.* (1999): 42 mixed, including teachers, nurses, social workers, psychologists (focused on reporting maltreatment of disabled children)

Focus	More likely to report if:
Child and family characteristics	• perception of maltreatment was high (Ashton, 2004) • there was strong evidence and concern for safety (Bryant and Milsom, 2005) • the children were in elementary rather than high school (Bryant and Milsom, 2005) • in schools where more children took free meals (Bryant and Milsom, 2005) • parents and children were white rather than African American (Hansen *et al.*, 1997) • children were younger (Hansen *et al.*, 1997)
Personal/ professional characteristics	• practitioner White and/or born in the US, Asian least likely (Ashton, 2004) • is less approving of corporal punishment (Ashton, 1999) • a social work practitioner with a personal history of maltreatment or domestic violence (Hansen *et al.*, 1997) • a psychologist with an existing professional history of reporting maltreatment (Hansen *et al.*, 1997)
System characteristics	• the law requires reporting (Bryant and Milsom, 2005) • there was less concern about the process of investigation (Bryant and Milsom, 2005) • previous reporting lead to a good outcome for a child (Mitchell *et al.*, 1999) • there was an absence of a range of system barriers (Mitchell *et al.*, 1999)

We were also interested in finding studies that took a wider view on response. In particular we were interested to explore what evidence existed about the direct provision of support to neglected children by a range of professions.

Professionals in the universal and voluntary services have long been concerned about thresholds for acceptance into the 'child protection system' (Department of Health 2002). This has been exacerbated by the way that the protective system has been preoccupied with forensic issues. There are questions as to whether this is the most appropriate way to ensure that neglected children receive help (Buckley 2005). A swathe of legislation and policy is now being rolled out in the UK that aims to remove the bottleneck effect of the mismatch between the need for support services and eligibility framed in terms of formal substantiation of 'neglect'. One of the aims is that the concept of thresholds should become less salient in a more integrated system where there is a collaborative assessment of needs and joint planning to meet unmet needs. There is also an expectation that universal services will provide direct support to neglected children. The *Getting it Right for Every Child* framework in Scotland states:

> Mainstream services (for example nurseries, schools, family centres, primary care services and youth centres) should be the front line providers of children's services. They should make sure children and their parents get the learning and support they need to do well. These front line providers of children's services are also the front line of support. Working in partnership with other agencies, they need to take early preventative measures. *Before referral to another service, agencies should take responsibility and do all they can, with the help of others, to support the child. The child should not automatically be passed to another agency.* (Scottish Executive 2005, p.11)

The evaluation of the early phases of the *Getting it Right for Every Child* pathfinder project in the Highlands is promising in that it does indicate that while child protection referrals and registrations were reduced, signs of child safety were increased and there was a clear focus on improving children's well-being (Stradling, MacNeil and Berry 2009). Structural changes such as bringing together the different types of assessment and planning meetings into one, and producing a single plan and identifying a lead professional all appear to have helped with streamlining the provision of support to children in the Highlands. In England the introduction of Local Safeguarding Children Boards (LSCBs) and Children's Trusts aimed to assist with more streamlined approaches to responding to children's needs (although subsequent policies may change some of these arrangements). An evaluation of LSCBs found that:

> Professionals at the strategic and operational levels are embracing
> the notion that safeguarding children is a shared responsibility,
> rather than one confined to Children's Social Care. However,
> there were differences of opinion as to whether LSCBs should
> be embracing the wider safeguarding agenda or concentrating
> their efforts more narrowly on protecting children from harm.
> (France, Munro and Waring 2010, p.i)

It was beyond the scope of this evaluation to look at outcomes for children,
but clearly more research to examine the impact on children of structural
strategic change is required.

Overall, therefore, the evidence base to support professionals (especially
those in universal services) to decide upon the most appropriate *response*
to a neglected child is still sparse. We would suggest that it is likely to be
of benefit for children if universal services are able to get on and provide
support for neglected children whether they are officially labelled as such or
not. But it is not surprising that there is still a lot of anxiety and confusion
about roles and responsibilities with regard to 'response'.

General public

An interesting, but sparsely covered line of research is systematic exploration
into whether members of the community would be prepared to take action,
and what form of action, if concerned about neglect. Some hints come from
a study of South Asian Canadians' views about levels of acceptable care
(Maiter, Alaggia and Trocme 2004). The study was limited to the views of
mothers and fathers who had immigrated to Canada during the previous
12 years from South Asia – no direct comparisons were made with the
indigenous population, but the authors suggest that their views about
acceptable care were not markedly different from the general population.
In focus groups respondents were asked to comment on help-seeking and
in one example 85.7 per cent thought it inappropriate to leave a six and
four-year-old alone whilst the parents were out late – 85.7 per cent said the
parents should get help, mainly from relatives/friends, although 27.8 per
cent said from social services. These respondents demonstrated the capacity
to identify neglect in the community, but – as the authors concluded –
'participants voiced their reluctance to contact child protective services
should they encounter families struggling with abuse' (p.309).

Andrews (1996) described a survey carried out as part of a public
awareness intiative in the US that focused on encouraging community
support for children of parents who misuse substances with a view to 'the
development of strong neighbourhoods where people care about, watch,

and support each others' families' (p.20). The underpinning theory to this approach is that people are more likely to seek and use help from those with whom they already have a relationship. In the survey of over 800 members of the public in a Southern state 89.1 per cent said they would help if they became aware of a child being abused or neglected as a result of parental substance misuse. However, the vast majority (86%) also stated that help would take the form of reporting the problem to formal agencies. Far fewer would offer more direct forms of help.

There are examples of public awareness raising campaigns that focus on encouraging members of the general public to report their concerns. The NSPCC *Full Stop* campaign, for example, provides information for the public on warning signs and on how to report (NSPCC 2011). The case study in Box 4.1 gives an example of the signs that prompted neighbours to raise concerns.

Box 4.1 Case study

Saskia is a single female carer. She is of White, British origin and she lives with her three children, who are all under eight years of age, in a town in the North of England. The children have different fathers, none of whom play active or meaningful parts in their lives. Saskia was in care herself as a child and she has little effective family support. She has experienced domestic violence. She is reliant upon benefits as her only source of income.

Saskia lives a transient lifestyle. She moves home frequently through privately rented accommodation which is paid for by housing benefit. In doing so, she frequently uproots her children physically, socially and educationally. One of the children attended three different reception classes, in three different schools, over the course of one academic year. When the children are enrolled at a school, their attendance, punctuality and attainment is poor. Legal action by the education directorate is being considered.

Through reports from neighbours, concerns increased substantially about the care that the children were receiving from their mother. Home conditions were hazardous as to the welfare and safety of the children. Doors were hanging off. The home stank of faeces and urine. There were not enough beds for the children to sleep in. Bedding was dirty and inadequate. There was little evidence of age appropriate toys, games or activities which could stimulate and assist the children in their enjoyment and development. Food was scarce and of low nutritional value.

The children's social presentation was very often dirty and unkempt. There were no effective routines or structure to their day. The children were reported to stay up into the early hours and arrive at school having had no breakfast. School also reported that the children came to school in dirty clothing and dirty underwear.

Saskia struggled to manage the children's behaviour effectively and appropriately. She failed to supervise them adequately. Within the family home, the children were reported to run riot; for example, they smeared faeces on the walls, deliberately urinated around the house and tried to start a fire in the living room. All of this set alarm bells sounding in more ways than one. The children had been exposed to severe domestic violence and although Saskia had ended her relationship with the perpetrator, there were concerns about a re-kindling of this relationship with the potential of further exposure of the children to severe physical and emotional harm.

Saskia persistently failed to attend to the routine health and medical needs of her children. She did not register the children with a GP despite two of the children having specific and significant health conditions which necessitated regular attendance and review with medical personnel.

Saskia latterly accepted a caution from police for criminal neglect due to failing to attend to one of her children's health needs and, as a result of this, she had caused permanent and avoidable damage to the child's health.

Due to the above, the children became subject to a child protection plan.

There are also examples of wider community involvement in providing a response beyond reporting. One would be the Children's Hearing system in Scotland where decisions about children who commit offences, and children who need care and protection are taken by Children's Panel members who are trained volunteers from the community (for more information see www.scra.gov.uk/home/index.cfm).

There is a good example of community involvement in the provision of direct support to children in England who are already subject to child protection plans. The Volunteers in Child Protection project (ViCP) trains and supports members of the community to provide direct support to both children and their parents. An evaluation of the pilot projects found that there were high levels of need in the families and that there were good levels of satisfaction with the personalized support that volunteers provided (Tunstill 2007). Tunstill notes the problems associated with the dominance of a narrow model of child protection within social services and suggests that it should be possible to provide such support without situations being formally identifed as child protection concerns. Drawing on the ecological model, Tunstill also suggests that there is need for more consideration of ways in which the community can be seen as a resource for families in need of support. These examples incorporate community resources within the structure of professional support and training. There is less information about ways in which the members of the community may provide informal support.

Health staff

The evidence on recognition suggested that health visitors are very well equipped to recognize the parental characteristics associated with neglect and the developmental signs in children. The most extensive evidence about *response* also related to the health profession and in particular health visitors. Eighty-six per cent of the Finnish hospital-based staff in Paavilainen *et al.*'s (2002) study said that when they suspect maltreatment they discuss it with the team of colleagues; 5 per cent that they refer to an outside agency (despite there being mandatory reporting legislation in Finland), 13 per cent that they discuss the concerns with the parents or child and 1 per cent that they do nothing. The researchers so effectively sum up the professional dilemma that it is worth quoting in full:

> Child maltreatment is such a difficult and sensitive issue that in order not to accuse innocent people the respondents wanted to be as sure as possible about a maltreatment case before they intervened. It is also such a distressing issue that it may be easier just to 'close one's eyes' to it than to investigate the case more thoroughly. The respondents were also doubtful about how to act and whether their interpretation was 'right' or whether suspicion was merely based on differing policy guidelines or cultural differences. Rareness and sensitivity of the phenomenon make it hard to intervene in child maltreatment cases – family is seen as something 'private' and it is largely thought that the way families raise their children is their own affair – the fear of offending families was great.' (p.293)

In relation to response in the UK, Appleton's study (1996) showed that 80 per cent of respondents saw themselves as referral agents, but many perceived the lack of social services resources as a barrier to referral and were '…angry and frustrated over the lack of social services input with families, particularly in those areas of "high concern" often described as "grey areas" (p.8). Similarly, in the US, English *et al.* (2005) found that a failure to provide basic needs, and caregivers' verbally aggressive behaviour were predictive of significant developmental delays as described previously. However, despite the potential for harm they observed that referrals of this nature did not always meet the organizations' defined thresholds of risk for substantiation.

Lagerberg's (2004) high quality Swedish study provides evidence about the actual referral practice of 1601 child health nurses. Between them 951 of the nurses noted that they were 'anxious' about a total of 6044 children, with the dominant concern being about 'disturbed parenting or neglect'. Despite the context of mandatory reporting in Sweden nurses were unlikely to have reported the children to social services and the rate of reporting of neglect was the lowest category of maletreatment at 8 per cent.

For children suspected as maltreated Thyen *et al.* (1997) found that medical practitioners were more likely to report concerns about infants than school-age children, and to refer in relation to the severity of the condition, for example, toxic ingestion or meningitis.

Health visitor anxieties often centre on what they should do as a result of their concerns because of their perception of high thresholds for access to services. The vision for health visiting in England *Facing the Future* (Lowe 2007) sets out two roles:

- leading and delivering the child health promotion programme using a family focused public health approach, or

- delivering intensive programmes for the most vulnerable children and families. (p.7)

This suggests a shift away from a model of referral on to social services for many situations where there may be early signs of potential neglect, towards a model of service delivery led by health visitors. Buckley's research (2005) suggested that this could be an effective approach. The evidence from the studies in our review about some role confusion and frustration at resource limitations suggests that considerable training and support will be required to ensure that health visitors can carry out both these roles effectively. The findings in Paavilainen *et al.*'s (2000) study offer an interesting model for a more active role for school nurses (see Box 4.2).

Box 4.2 Research highlight

Paavilainen, E., Astedt-Kurki, P. and Paunonen, M. (2000) 'School nurses' operational modes and ways of collaborating in caring for child abusing families in Finland.' *Journal of Clinical Nursing, 9,* 5, 742–750.

Paavilainen *et al.* undertook a study on the role of school nurses in order to explain and conceptualize the working methods used by them when caring for child abusing families.

In Finland children start school at age 7. All children have regular check-ups by school nurses for vision, growth, hearing, etc., and relationships between health conditions and school performance are monitored. This work offers opportunities for both identifying concerns, and planning and implementing care. School nurses have a legal obligation to report detections of child abuse to the child protection authorities.

Semi-structured interviews were held with 20 Finnish school nurses representing between them a diversity of schools and experiences. The interviews were transcribed verbatim and analysed using inductive techniques.

All school nurses had experience of children whose school performance had suffered as a result of maltreatment. Paavilainen *et al.* found two kinds of working: an active and firm mode and a passive and uninvolved mode.

Active and firm mode

If a school nurse suspected abuse, they would begin to gather more information about the family (they called this 'detective work'):

> The school nurse's main aim was to act in a way that solved problems in favour of the child... These nurses knew their clients and were interested in developing their work on a continuous basis with child abusing families. Active and firm school nurses were not afraid of interfering and did not wait needlessly, expecting things to turn out right by themselves. (p.742)

The active and firm mode nurses would immediately involve the family and used a rather no-nonsense approach. As one nurse explained:

> 'I had a phone call saying that the children had spent the night unattended at home. I told the parents straightforwardly that I had had a call. I asked them what they are doing, how can a thing like this happen. We discussed the matter... and we

agreed what to do. I make regular house calls, I am not going to leave them on their own... I just pop in now and then... So far they have not thrown me out once.' (p.743)

Passive and uninvolved mode

Not all the school nurses had such a working model however. The passive and uninvolved would immediately hand over to other professional groups working with the families. They felt overwhelmed by the enormity and complexity of child protection cases and felt there was no point in tackling the problems 'as there wasn't much you could do about it'. Unless absolutely certain of maltreatment, they preferred to wait and see what would happen:

'I've tried to do something at least in some serious cases... It didn't work out, it's no use. You must handle the client discreetly or they won't come anymore. So as not to hurt their feelings.' (p.744)

Education staff

The lack of empirical evidence about the role of schools is concerning given the centrality placed on schools in England in *The Children's Plan*:

Almost all children, young people and families come into regular contact with early years settings and with schools and colleges. That means early years settings, schools and colleges must sit at the heart of an effective system of prevention and early intervention working in partnership with parents and families... If these services are not integrated with more specialist provision, by looking for early warnings that children might need more help and by providing facilities for specialist services to operate so they can be easily reached by children and families, we will be hamstrung in achieving our broad ambitions for children and young people. (DCSF 2007a, p.144)

Following a survey of initial teacher education in England that showed considerable variation in the quality of child protection coverage, a course was developed by the NSPCC for student teachers and evaluated by Baginsky (2000; 2003). Although the teachers had valued the training they were troubled by the disparity between what they had learned about good practice in relation to referral and their actual experiences in schools. They had heard colleagues questioning the value of making referrals to social services and they expressed a lot of confusion about neglect. Based on their training they could identify neglect but were advised by schools that these children would be unlikely to be defined as 'neglected'. On the basis of a follow-up survey Baginsky (2003) recommends the need for ongoing training.

In Australia there are mandatory reporting laws, but teachers are still confused about their roles. Laskey (2008) identified a number of factors that affect willingness to make referrals including anxiety, lack of training and a lack of confidence in the system to make things better for the child (including from those who had previous experience of making referrals). Teachers wanted and sought support from colleagues to discuss their concerns despite strict confidentiality requirements.

Webster *et al.*'s study (2005) focuses more on abuse but considers the issue of under- or over-reporting in the context of mandatory reporting laws in Ohio. They discuss the debate about whether we should be more concerned about over-reporting of abuse or under-reporting of abuse and describe it as 'a major social policy controversy' (p.1282).

In order to find out what variables affect under-and-over reporting 480 teachers rated 24 vignettes combining 9 variables describing a potential child abuse event. Teachers rated each vignette on two scales – 'not child abuse' to 'child abuse' (recognition) and 'unlikely to report' to 'likely to report' (response). In 62.6 per cent of the total number of vignettes scored the teacher scores for recognition and response were equal (consistent reporting). In 4.2 per cent the reporting score was higher than the recognition score (over-reporting) while in 33.2 per cent the response scores were lower than the recognition scores (under-reporting).

These findings suggest a tendency towards under-reporting rather than over-reporting. Consistent reporting was seen to be associated with cases that were seen to be more serious or unambiguous, especially sexual abuse. Where cases were seen to be less serious or more ambiguous teachers tended to use more discretion about reporting, or rather – not reporting. Teacher characteristics associated with under-reporting included beliefs that reporting would cause problems for the teacher or child and not having reported an incident in the past. There are implications here for neglect – neglect is certainly often ambiguous and is frequently viewed as less serious that other forms of maltreatment.

Taken as a whole it is reasonable to expect that there is considerable under-reporting of neglect by teachers. Teachers do see it as their responsibility to look out for the welfare of children and are not unwilling to help, but there are clearly concerns and anxieties about 'the system' and these appear to be especially acute with regard to neglect. Teachers cannot operate in a vacuum – there needs to be a local multi-disciplinary context of trust and respect, coupled with good support at school level if teachers are to feel confident about responding to the signs that they see in their classrooms.

There is little research about the potential role of schools in directly ameliorating the impact of neglect. In a very small, but insightful study based on interviews with four teachers, Maggiolo (1998) describes ways in which teachers can provide an 'island of safety for neglected children' (p.4) by helping them to develop self-control and self-worth, by acknowledging their feelings and offering opportunities for choices and exploration. She concludes:

> Teachers will encounter cases of neglect throughout their teaching years and it is important to help these children gain more self-esteem and positive feelings of being appreciated, loved, and valued by others. Even though it is our job to report these cases, it should also be in our hearts to help. Just think, if it wasn't for someone who noticed, it might have continued forever. (p.12)

Baginsky's edited book (2008) gives many policy, practice and training suggestions about how schools can promote the health and welfare of children, establish a protective ethos and provide support for children with a range of additional needs.

Social workers

The evidence about the social work/social services early response is rather minimal and tends to focus on investigation and assessment. In a well-known UK study of practice with 712 referrals to social services because of child protection concerns or the need for a service, Wilding and Thoburn (1997) showed that concerns about neglect were given less priority and acted on 39 per cent of the time compared with an average of 70 per cent for physical or sexual abuse. The pattern continued as cases of neglect were less likely to be taken to case conference or the children registered, and families tended to be steered away from services.

Generally, there was agreement in the studies on the characteristics identified as significant in the substantiation of neglect: children were more vulnerable, fragile and had more challenging or difficult behaviour and were less likely to be protected (Scannapieco and Connell-Carrick 2005).

As Stevenson (1998) suggested, knowledge of the limitations of the alternatives and a tendency to become inured to neglect can affect professional judgement. There may be merit in ensuring that the process of assessing whether a child's needs are not being met for whatever reason is clearly separated from decisions about how best to respond. The evidence suggests that a preoccupation with matters such as parental culpability and whether statutory measures are required can obscure the initial careful assessment as to whether any needs are unmet and can affect thresholds for recognition. In other words, it could be helpful for practice if thresholds for recognition of unmet need could be disentangled from the thresholds for application of the 'official' definition of neglect (Daniel 2005).

Since Wilding's research there has been far more attention to the impact of neglect upon children and recent statistics indicate that neglect has been the leading category for children being made subject to child protection plans in England in each year from 2006–2010 (Department for Education 2010). For many children and families workers the majority of their work is with neglect. Even if neglect has not been the primary cause for allocation, it is often the backdrop for more acute concerns. A considerable amount of social work effort is, therefore, directed towards improving the lives of neglected children. The fact that other professionals are still frustrated by the numbers of children they notice who need additional help but do not receive it underlines the need for a multi-disciplinary response. It also highlights the need for more prevention and early intervention – issues that are addressed in Chapter 6.

Improving recognition and response

The majority of studies identified training as the solution to improving recognition and response. However, there has been very little systematic research into the impact of training on recognition and reporting (Ogilvie-Whyte 2006); see also Carpenter's study (Carpenter *et al.* 2010). Only two studies that met the criteria for our review focused on training. Narayan *et al.*'s study (2006) suggested that physician preparedness to address child abuse and neglect at qualification from paediatric training in the States was related to the extent and quality of direct teaching and involvement in mandatory clinical rotations in child abuse and neglect. This study was limited to self-report and there was no measurement of actual recognition or reporting behaviour.

In a high-quality study, Angeles Cerezo and Pons-Salvador (2004) indicated that, with the right conditions, response could be swifter and more accurate. They undertook a comprehensive two-phase intervention study in an area of Spain that focused both on recognition and response (albeit reporting) and did measure behaviour. In phase one 181 professionals representing all the relevant agencies in the area from social services, police and health (medical, nursing, psychology and psychiatry) were trained in child protection. In the second phase, over the following two years 251 professionals from schools, including teachers, psychologists and pedagogues were trained. The team undertook considerable preparatory work in devising referral forms and referral processes. Throughout the intervention period a local coordination team was in place to offer flexible support, guidance and consultation to agencies and professionals. The findings were impressive: following the first phase detection tripled from 0.58 to 1.77 per 1000 children.

Following the introduction of training in schools, the detection rate again increased to 2.18 per 1000 children – of the new cases 24.5 per cent could be directly attributed to reporting from schools. Significantly, the confirmation rate moved from 43 per cent before the intervention to 88 per cent afterwards which means that recognition was more accurate. The authors especially emphasize the role of teachers:

> Our results showed that the program increased detection in schools after providing training and on-line support to school professionals. The specific intervention addressed their fears and doubts about what would be best for the child and also their lack of confidence and knowledge on their contribution regarding the protection of children… the results of this study showed that there is a unique and relevant role for schools. (p.1166)

The evidence about the barriers, such as those set out in Table 4.1, supports the importance of developing more effective integrated approaches to children where all professions regard themselves as part of the child well-being system. The evidence also suggests that protocols and guidelines are not a sufficient spur to response. Human issues such as trust, relationships, communication, anxiety, fear and confidence affect willingness to act on concerns. Angeles Cerezo and Pons-Salvador (2004) attribute the success of their study to the fact that they built in a mechanism to provide ongoing support, advice and guidance to professionals to complement the huge training initiative. The concept of the 'space for negotiation' as described by Cooper *et al.* (2003) allows for the fact that issues such as child neglect are rarely concrete – they are complex, multifaceted and merit discussion.

Assessment and planning

There is a dilemma in how to deal with assessment, because assessment is not a discrete, middle phase of the chronology of helping. Assessment is happening at all stages. All of us are making minute-by-minute assessments of those around us all of the time. When encountering any child a mass of conscious or unconscious judgements are made about the way the child is dressed, behaves, how they relate to us or others and so on. All sorts of relative comparisons are made against all sorts of internal rulers. The early stages of noticing that something may be awry with a child will be guided by this mixed bag and it is more helpful to practitioners to recognize that it is as much their humanity as their professionalism that will influence early recognition (Helm 2010). If matters progress, and the child becomes subject to more formal proceedings, then informal assessment morphs into the more formally defined system processes of 'initial assessment' and 'comprehensive assessment'. At these stages it is important not to let the process become mystified or overly-complex. Rigour and structure are important in assessment and planning, but they should not be equated with rigidity and inflexibility. Here we will examine some of the factors that need to be taken into account when undertaking multi-disciplinary assessments as the basis for service delivery to help a neglected child. The key question throughout the assessment process is:

- What does this child and their family or carer need me to think about?

Theory for assessment

Based on the studies described, especially in Chapter 2, the ecological model is confirmed as a powerful framework for locating the range of factors that can signal the potential for neglect. Such a model takes account of environment, culture, structures and different levels of support (psychological, sociological and material) that can enhance or detract from care. The significance of parental past experiences indicates the need to apply the ecological framework to past as well as to present events. The *Framework for Assessment* (Department of Health 1999) does include 'Family history and functioning' – but the evidence suggests that the complete ecological framework should be applied to any assessment of families, including both past and present indicators that may have compromised adequate parenting, or could be strengthened to avoid harm.

The ecological-transactional-developmental framework recognizes that development is a dynamic process shaped by interactions between environment, caregiver and child as well as interactions of previous experience with current functioning (Brandon *et al.* 2008). It takes account of individual, family, social and structural factors affecting development and the relationship histories of parents and the quality of children's attachments.

Knowledge of attachment theory is also especially helpful in neglect cases. A superficial understanding of attachment theory can be dangerous because in neglect cases anxious attachments are often misinterpreted as strong bonds to be preserved at all costs. Howe *et al.* (1999)'s work provides an accessible but comprehensive model for a more nuanced analysis of the range of attachment patterns that may develop in the context of different types of neglectful relationships. A broader understanding of relationships and especially the power of an effective working or therapeutic relationship between practitioners and parents and children is also important. There has been a resurgence of attention to the relationship aspect of practice (see Howe 2008). We return to this in more depth in the next chapter. An understanding of relationships can assist with effective multi-disciplinary practice, where the quality of the overall support for children can depend on the quality of the protective network. Coupled with a basic knowledge of child development, especially the key developmental tasks occurring at each stage, these theories will support comprehensive assessment and planning.

Multi-disciplinary assessment and planning

Very rarely will a neglected child's needs be of relevance to one profession only. Sometimes there may be a very specific form of neglect, for example, a child may be well-nourished, healthy and active but not encouraged to attend school. Another may have all their needs met except the need for dental treatment. However, the majority of children who are neglected are experiencing a constellation of unmet need and their parents are affected by a constellation of challenges and problems. Assessment and planning with neglect, therefore, will pretty much always require the input from all key professions and a number of other agencies and relevant parties.

The Graded Care Profile (GCP) provides a helpful framework for assessment where there are concerns about neglect (Svrivastava *et al.* 2003). Health visitors and social workers are often trained together in the use of the GCP and this supports mutual understanding and a common language for comprehensive assessment. The GCP can be used in conjunction with existing broad assessment frameworks.

Together the different agencies need to be involved in assessing:

- the child's unmet needs in all domains
- the reasons for needs not being met

- parental capacity to meet those needs
- parental motivation to meet the child's needs with support
- parental capacity to adapt and change with support
- whether compulsory measures might be required.

Unmet needs

Evidence-based frameworks for practice offer structure to help with assessing each domain of a child's life. The English model will be familiar to many and covers the key dimensions of children's development. The Scottish model (see Figure 4.2) is similar, but helpful because it is set out from the child's perspective. And it is absolutely vital to gain the child's views and feelings and to involve the children as far as possible in the assessment and planning process.

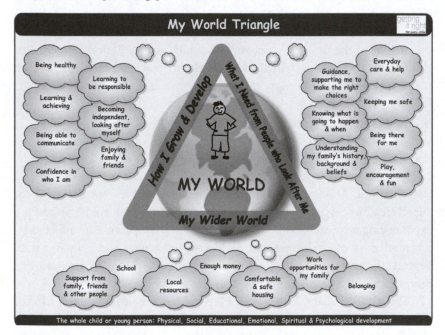

Figure 4.2: Showing the 'My World' triangle, part of the Scottish *Getting it Right for Every Child* model (Scottish Executive 2005)

What the ecological-transactional-developmental model reminds us is that, although it is important to consider each side of the triangle, it is also important to consider interactions. So, for example, 'understanding my family's history, background and beliefs' could impact upon 'confidence in who I am'. And 'comfortable and safe housing' can impact upon 'being healthy'. All domains should be considered for all children, children with additional needs – perhaps as a result of disability – are as entitled to a full life as all children.

Information about each domain should be collated on the basis of the expertise of all the professionals involved. Chapter 2 illustrated just how many aspects of a child's development can be affected by neglect. Information from direct observation of children in different contexts and children with their parents is invaluable. The implications for development of a need remaining unmet can then be extrapolated. At this stage there may be a necessity for some immediate planning to address urgent unmet need – for example, if a child requires treatment for a serious health condition, is seriously undernourished, or is in danger from contact with risky adults. But detailed planning for the longer term will not be complete without fuller assessment.

Reasons for unmet need

This issue overlaps very much with issues of parental capacity, but it is helpful to consider all possible reasons for needs not being met. For example, there may be undiagnosed medical issues – deafness may be affecting learning, illness may be affecting growth, bullying may be affecting confidence, a poor or failing school may be affecting learning and so on. Plans to address neglect should incorporate attention to any issues such as these.

Parental capacity to meet needs

As shown in Chapter 3 parenting capacity is frequently undermined by substance misuse, domestic violence and mental health problems. As far as possible, it is important to assess the quality of parenting when not intoxicated. This will affect the intervention plan, if parenting when not intoxicated is reasonable then the focus should be primarily on addressing the substance misuse; if parenting is lacking when not intoxicated, then there will need to be attention to underlying knowledge and skills of parenting. Assessment and the subsequent plan must be very explicit about how factors affecting parenting capacity will be addressed. In a study of a cohort of neglected children who had been removed from home and later returned it was found that:

> In half (51%) of the cases a clear focus on important issues in the case had not been maintained at times by children's social care services and in a considerable number of families key problems had not been addressed, in particular parental alcohol and drugs misuse, domestic violence, mental health problems and lack of parenting skills. (Farmer and Lutman 2010, p.2)

If needs in some domains are being met it is also worth understanding why. There may be aspects of capacity that could be transferred to other domains. Again, it is crucial to involve both parents and any other important adults in the process of assessment and planning. 'Working in partnership' is easy to suggest, but it is important to acknowledge that it can be especially challenging in cases of neglect. But efforts to establish relationships with important adults will not be wasted. Even if it proves almost impossible to establish some kind of connection, this is valuable information.

Parental motivation

Horwath and Morrison's model (2001) for exploring capacity and willingness to change remains the most helpful for assessing parental motivation to change and to change within a quick enough timeframe to match the child's developmental trajectory. The model comprises two dimensions – one of levels of effort and one of levels of commitment. When these are combined there are four possible categories:

1. 'Genuine commitment' where parents make good efforts to change and show commitment to improving their parenting for the benefit of the children.

2. 'Tokenism' where parents express commitment to change, but for a range of possible reasons do not put in actual effort to change.

3. 'Compliance imitation' or 'approval seeking' where there can be high effort to make changes (perhaps sporadically) but the commitment to sustained change is not demonstrated.

4. 'Dissent' or 'avoidance' where there is a combination of low effort and low commitment.

It may take some time to assess these dimensions: however, children or their families have often been known to professionals for a long time and careful scrutiny of past patterns of response to support should give helpful insights into motivation to change. There are dangers in waiting too long to establish motivation to change. On the basis of assessment of motivation, practitioners, when making their plans, should ask themselves whether they are succumbing to the 'start-again' syndrome where parents are given too many chances with successive children to change (Brandon *et al.* 2008).

Parental capacity to adapt and change

Neglected children are often described as living in complex families, which somehow implies that others families are not complex. These families are also often described as hard to change, but such terms can be unhelpful. The label of 'hard to change' is, of course, aiming to articulate concepts that will be familiar to many practitioners, and it would be naïve to suggest that the concept does not have some validity. The problem is that it can be used to explain away lack of effective practice to improve the child's life and can be used to locate the blame for lack of progress with parents. It springs from the frustration and anxiety that goes with the territory of working with people with the characteristics described in Chapter 3.

What is surprising is the extent to which some of these characteristics seem to be surprising to the practitioner network, because they are the very factors that combine to create and exacerbate neglect in the first place. Standing back from simple labels and identifying, assessing and tackling the characteristics that manifest as hard to reach or hard to change would be a very helpful starting point for planning effective intervention. It would also be very helpful for practitioners to be able to recognize the feelings that these characteristics provoke. Working to improve neglected children's lives can be sapping; the sense of hopelessness that parents often feel about their situation can be transmitted to practitioners and it can be very difficult to maintain one's own optimism in the face of unremitting pessimism (Daniel 1999a). To avoid succumbing to a cycle of hopelessness it is helpful to have the opportunity to stand back and reflect upon the dynamic of the working relationship – something that can be assisted with good supervision, consultation or peer support. It could also be helpful to take some time to consider what kind of messages the children are gathering about life from a climate of pessimism (see Box 4.3).

Box 4.3 Activity

Labels such as hard to reach and hard to change may spring from the frustration and anxiety that goes with the territory of working with people who exhibit a range of characteristics. But it is these characteristics that are often the root of the problem – they combine to create and exacerbate neglect in the first place. Assessment and planning is more effective if practitioners can stand back from labels and instead identify, assess and plan to address the characteristics that manifest as hard to reach or hard to change. It is important to recognize the feelings that these characteristics provoke in practitioners, but also in members of the community who may have tried to offer support and help.

1. Consider the parental characteristics below.
2. Add any others that you have encountered.
3. Think about how easily labels can be applied to parents.
4. Stand back from the characteristics and think about how and why they are associated with neglect.
5. Think about what a plan aimed at addressing these issues head-on would look like.
6. Consider the impact upon practitioners and what can be put in place to avoid the erosion of self-efficacy that ripples through the helping network.

Many parents of neglected children:

- avoid contact with professionals
- appear not to recognize that there is anything wrong with their children's development
- keep repeating patterns of behaviour that apparently make them and/or their children unhappy
- stick with partners or family members whose behaviour is violent, cruel or undermining
- say they will do something and then do not do it
- exhibit behaviour and language that is abusive, obstructive or dismissive
- miss meetings, forget arrangements or arrive intoxicated
- become pregnant swiftly after one child has been removed from their care
- promise to attend specialist services but do not go to them
- represent the second or third generation in a family which has been subject to similar professional concerns about childcare
- go over and over the same details of their past and seem never to be able to move beyond them
- seem to have no energy, no hope, no optimism and seem unable to visualize any kind of positive future.

KEY MESSAGES

1. The research on recognition suggests that signs are often obvious to members of the community and their concerns need to be heard.

2. Professionals need to ensure that their involvement with systems, professional constraints and bureaucracy do not blinker them to the needs of neglected children.

3. Health visitors should continue to draw upon their clinical and assessment skills when working with parents with young children rather than seek the false reassurance of predictive checklists.

4. Intuitive awareness can play an important role in recognition that things may not be right for a child.

5. Health staff are in a key position to notice medical and non-medical signs of incipient neglect.

6. Practitioners should be alert to the factors that might be blocking their willingness to act on their concerns about children and seek to overcome them with support and training.

7. There is a need to build on the evidence about the skills health visitors have in recognition, in combination with research into the most effective immediate and longer-term response.

8. The 'active and firm mode' as practised by some Finnish school nurses offers an interesting model to consider.

9. Policy that places schools at the heart of early intervention must acknowledge that there is a paucity of evidence about the most effective way for this role to be undertaken.

10. Practice frameworks should ensure that the process of integrated initial assessment of children's needs is separated from decisions about action required to ensure needs are met.

5

Helping the Neglected Child

Introduction

Previous chapters have considered the terms and language used to describe neglect; how families and children signal, directly and indirectly, their concerns about neglect; and in what ways professionals recognize and respond to neglect. This chapter considers the research evidence regarding what works and who works in supporting children and families to prevent neglect escalating and to ameliorate the effects of neglect. The research discussed in this chapter is not drawn primarily from our systematic literature review because it did not focus on interventions. However, we have drawn on Moran's (2009) review undertaken for Action for Children and a range of wider literature on interventions.

Having said that, the literature is in fact relatively sparse in relation to what works in situations where a child or young person has been maltreated, and the term *neglect* is often conflated with other forms of *abuse* (Barlow and Schrader-Macmillan 2009; Montgomery *et al.* 2009). Tanner and Turney (2006) succinctly summarize the shortcomings in the evidence base concerning effective interventions:

- a reliance on studies from the US whose findings may not necessarily transfer to a UK context
- a variation in the way that neglect is defined, including the scope of what is included in the definition
- the failure to distinguish between neglect and abuse, with interventions tending to be aimed at vulnerable families where either or both neglect and abuse may be occurring

- a lack of theoretical basis or else theoretical basis not being explicitly stated, aside from the ecological model or other models drawn from psychology, child development but rarely social work

- a lack of attention to the way in which interventions address issues of ethnicity, gender, class and culture, and

- methodological shortcomings such as small sample sizes, or differences in outcome measures.

Thoburn (2009) undertook a review of effective practice in working with children and families at risk of significant harm. The review concluded that no single service approach or method had yet been identified to be effective with families where the concerns of harm were significant and complex. Instead, such interventions were likely to represent one part of an overall package required to support families experiencing difficulties. Moran (2009) comments that few interventions specifically target neglect. Some interventions are designed to improve outcomes for disadvantaged children, young people and families in general rather than being designed specifically for, and targeted at families where the children are neglected. The interventions are often aimed at 'high risk' families in which neglect and child maltreatment are likely to be at elevated rates, and tackle factors that are thought to contribute to neglect.

Barlow with Scott (2010) comment that, while there are no easy answers about what works, the evidence does provide important indications about the key elements of practice that are necessary for effective working. This concurs with Moran's (2009) review in which it was argued that the characteristics of interventions that are most likely to succeed could be drawn from evidence of what appears to be 'promising' and pertinent in cases of neglect, given its chronic, complex nature; and from the significance of ecological and attachment models for understanding its causes.

Another emergent theme from the literature is the importance of therapeutic relationships and that 'who works' is as important as 'what works'. This points to the need for experienced practitioners who are skilled in the ability to develop relationships with children, families and other professionals; and who have also the ability to retain empathy for the family while not losing sight of the child and continued risks of neglect. Practitioners undertaking skilled casework also require good clinical supervision to provide space for both reflection and emotional support.

In this chapter we consider the principles of intervention that can be identified and examine what research tells us about interventions. The underpinning question for practitioners in this chapter is:

- What does this child and their family or carer need me to do?

Principles of intervention

Some principles of intervention that can be commonly identified suggest that it should:

- incorporate relationship building and attachment
- be long-term rather than episodic
- be multifaceted
- be offered early as well as late
- consider both protective and risk factors
- involve fathers or male caregivers as well as female caregivers.

Relationship building and attachment

At the heart of any intervention is a need to move from a focus on shared communication to a focus on shared *expertise*. This includes what parents and carers can offer, in order to ensure that all children can access the universal services of health, education and leisure. The accumulated evidence confirms that a range of factors can impact upon parenting capacity, but as previous chapters have identified, parents are able to identify concerns about themselves as parents (Combs-Orme *et al.* 2004) and the impact of their actions and behaviours upon their children (McKeganey *et al.* 2002). Professionals working with adults need to recognize that paying attention to the parenting role will enhance their practice with the adults themselves:

> An understanding of the impact of parenting can be enormously valuable to AOD [alcohol and other drug] workers. It can improve your drug treatment outcomes and help prevent cycles of inter-generational problems.
>
> For AOD workers, discussing a client's parental responsibilities and stresses can be crucial in assessing and responding to their drug problems. It's part of good drug treatment. (Burke and Gruenert 2005, p.1)

Research (Cowan and Cowan 2008) has identified the importance of family relationships in terms of the risk presented to children; attachment relationships are one route for a parent's past experience to impact on a child's development. The suggestion is that parents who provide harmful parenting in terms of their child's development may have been exposed to environments that did not meet their needs in their own childhoods. This can result in difficulties for these adults in responding to signals from their children (Barlow with Scott 2010). The relationship with, and quality of, a practitioner's response to a family's needs can help families address emotional difficulties and develop parental capacity to parent a child.

Given the significance of attachment issues as a framework for linking many of the factors contributing to neglect, interventions that draw on attachment theory as their basis are likely to be important for intervening with families where children are neglected. Secure attachment is a protective factor; hence enabling its development within children and also parents is likely to increase the probability of better child and family outcomes. In a discussion of attachment-based interventions for working with families in cases of neglect and abuse, Howe (2005) cites four different points of focus for interventions. These involve:

1. enhancing parents' sensitivity and responsiveness to their infant by changing parenting behaviour

2. changing parents' working model/mental representation of relationships through increasing insight and reflective capacity

3. providing enhanced social support for parents, and

4. improving maternal mental health and well-being.

When parents and carers experience attachment difficulties in relationships, it is likely that they may also experience difficulties in their relationships with agencies that are attempting to intervene. Parents' feelings of mistrust and of being blamed can reduce the success of an intervention, and such feelings are often present in their dealings with practitioners from services. Professionals need to be skilled in working empathically, respectfully, and in *partnership with* families rather than being seen as doing things *to* families (Forehand and Kotchik 2002). Practice should be based around an approach that is open and non-collusive and looks at a variety of interventions to help the whole family.

Intervention from statutory services in particular can be experienced as a threat to parents or carers. Buckley (2005) suggests that services offered by agencies outside the statutory system may be seen as more 'friendly', and can form part of a package of support if there are clear lines of accountability and contracting arrangements.

The skilful use of relationships to achieve outcomes for children can also be achieved if practitioners take time to discover the inner world of the child and what is significant to them in their own lives.

Long-term rather than episodic

Neglect is often chronic in nature, involving a complex interplay of entrenched family difficulties. It is crucial to look back as well as forward to improve long-term relationships within the family. There is not likely to be a quick fix remedy available. Therefore services working with families where children are neglected must recognize the need to work with some families on a long-term basis. Long-term professional commitment may also contribute to the building of more secure family attachments. Tanner and Turney (2003) recognize the value of families having long-term relationships with services as a means of offering parents an alternative model of attachment and a way of relating, although 'dysfunctional' dependency also needs to be recognized (Horwath 2007). Therefore, some of the elements that can be addressed in a long-term relationship include:

- *modelling*: assisting people to establish and maintain satisfactory interpersonal relationships

- *practicalities*: an understanding of the client's daily lived experience enables the relationship between client and professional to be used to engage with some of the more practical difficulties experienced by families

- *managed dependence*: interventions and plans that build in the concept of managed dependence aim to avoid both the start-again and revolving door syndromes.

'Managed dependence' is a concept coined by Tanner and Turney (2003) to capture the need for sustained approaches to support for parents. Rather than trying to 'move people to independence' it can be more fruitful to expect that support will be required over the long term and to plan accordingly. This is not to be equated with drifting packages of care where many resources are piled into a situation but without appreciable improvements for the child. All parents are dependent, to a greater or lesser extent, on additional support throughout their lives. But some families require more. In many cases parents can provide sufficient care for their children as long as they know they can rely on consistent additional support that will not be withdrawn the moment there are small signs of improvement. Perversely the fear of removal of services can act as a disincentive to change.

The application of effective interventions is complex and one intervention strategy is unlikely to succeed with all families where neglect of children is an issue. Long-term support aimed towards increasing self-esteem and independence, and provision of a supportive albeit challenging relationship are key features in overcoming neglect. These approaches are supported by research and find effective fruition in practice. The challenge for policy-makers is to enable there to be adequate funding for long-term support services to work alongside shorter, sharper, focused interventions so that change is made and is sustained through support for the most vulnerable parents and neediest families.

Multi-faceted

Given the long list of factors potentially contributing to neglect, approaches are required that intervene at multiple levels, influencing individual, family and social systems. Interventions are therefore more likely to succeed if they are multifaceted, tackling multiple risk factors. Packages of care may include a combination of interventions addressing a range of needs such as mental health issues and parenting skills as well as increasing social support and housing needs.

Multifaceted interventions can be shaped round a chronic problem, which may have existed in the family for many years. Intervention can also be a linear process. It is often the case that, when a family is referred for support due to one apparent issue, a rapport develops with the professional involved, leading to a multitude of issues emerging. What is needed is flexibility on behalf of both the worker and the service, so that multiple and cross-cutting issues are addressed, based on an understanding of the history of problems leading to the neglect.

Neglect is multifaceted in individual cases. Attending only to the practical or psychological aspects of neglect is only one part of a response. Multiagency integrated working by professionals is key to ensure all aspects of neglect receive attention, and to challenge whether interventions are making a difference. Asking all professions to work together *does not* mean everyone trying to do everyone else's job or everyone becoming a 'child protection' worker. But it *does* mean:

- creating the conditions that will allow children to benefit from the core service that each profession offers

- ensuring that *all* children get access to health care, education, social and emotional support – whatever the level of parental capacity

- developing services that are accessible to parents and children.

Early as well as late

Interventions can be described as 'early' or 'late' both in relation to the timing of the intervention relative to a child's age and in relation to the stage in development of the problem to be addressed. In relation to children's age, there is a need for intervention across childhood, as neglect can occur at any time from infancy to teenage years (Horwath 2007). There is also a need for intervention in infancy and before three years of age, given what is known about brain development and quality of caregiving. Whatever the chronological age of the child involved, the child's developmental age needs to be taken into account when designing interventions, as indeed, does the parents' (Howe 2005).

Protective and risk factors

Interventions also need to consider how to bolster individual and family strengths and resources in order to build child and adult resilience. It has been suggested that providing opportunities for the development of protective factors can reduce the likelihood of succumbing to the impact of adverse childhood experiences (Garbarino, Vorrasi and Kostelny 2002). In relation to neglect, as described earlier, providing opportunities to develop supportive relationships is important, and may have influence in building secure attachments and enhancing self-worth and self-efficacy. Horwath (2007) suggests provision of a support figure in cases of neglect, and this can arise from a positive childcare, nursery or school environment where staff may provide for the emotional and social needs of the child.

Involve fathers as well as mothers

Parenting interventions often fail to take into account that parents can be male as well as female (Moran, Ghate and van der Merwe 2004). Neglect in particular is an area where the role of mothers has been the focus of attention to the exclusion of men. As Daniel and Taylor (2005) point out, this unfortunate exclusion of fathers from the issue of neglect '...ignores the potential risks that men can pose to children and also misses the opportunity to build on what fathers and paternal extended families may offer children' (p.263). Box 5.1 gives an example of involving both parents.

Box 5.1 Case study

Background

Annie is 18 months old and of White Scottish origin. She lives with her mother, Daisy (21) and her father, Jimmy (22) in temporary accommodation in a deprived area within a central Scottish town. Their flat is cramped, poorly furnished and cluttered. Daisy was adopted as an infant herself and is estranged from her adoptive family. Jimmy is from a large local family and is the oldest of six children. There were concerns about Jimmy during his childhood due to domestic abuse and over chastisement of Jimmy and his siblings.

The child

Annie is underweight and small for her age. She has dark circles under her eyes, her face is pale and her hair is thin. Her nails are overgrown and dirty. Annie has little speech and is not meeting her developmental milestones. She is often dressed in the same stained babygro for days on end. Annie always seems to have nappy rash, caused by insufficient nappy changes and poor hygiene. Daisy finds it difficult to attend to Annie's needs and ignores her when she seeks comfort and proximity. Annie presents as a listless, sad child. There are no toys for her to play with and she is often put into her cot for long periods when she is being 'difficult'.

The response

Annie's poor condition was discovered when her parents took her to hospital with severe diarrhoea. The casualty doctor admitted Annie and referred her to duty social work. The social worker, Jenny, meets with Daisy and Jimmy in the hospital to discuss the concerns for Annie. Although initially worried and hostile, Daisy and Jimmy eventually express a sense of relief that support may be available to them. Jimmy says he is worried by Annie's poor health and Daisy says that she sometimes feels Annie hates her as she often won't eat food she has prepared and she screams when Daisy changes her nappy. They both agree to participate in a programme of assessment and support.

Jenny's initial assessment indicates that there are three main areas that the family need support on – practical support in caring for Annie, understanding and promoting Annie's physical and emotional development and considering their own experiences of being parented and forming attachments. Jenny organizes a core group meeting to coordinate the support to Annie and her family and an intensive support plan is agreed. An experienced early years practitioner visits the family twice per week and works with them on the priority issues of nutrition, hygiene and stimulation. She facilitates Daisy and Jimmy attending a special parent-toddler group with Annie where they learn how to play and interact more appropriately with her. The health visitor visits weekly to weigh Annie and provide advice on promoting Annie's development.

Jenny organizes separate visits each week with Jimmy and Daisy to explore and consider their experiences of being parented using an adult attachment perspective. It becomes clear that Daisy's early experience of disruption of attachments is impacting on her ability to form an attachment with Annie. As work progresses, Daisy better understands that Annie's reluctance to have her nappy changed, for example, stems from it being a painful experience for her, not because she is rejecting Daisy. By working with Daisy to reduce her negative attributions of Annie and with both parents to give them confidence in meeting Annie's needs, the situation gradually improves. This is evidenced by Annie gaining weight, developing more speech, becoming more animated and presenting as a much healthier, happier child.

Child-focused interventions

Some interventions involve working with children in addition to parents, but relatively little has been documented concerning direct work with children that specifically targets the impact of neglect, and there is even less that has been adequately evaluated. While parents who neglect their children clearly need support to enable them to provide a sufficiently nurturing environment for their children, children also need direct services in their own right. Interventions targeting children are usually aimed at helping the child overcome the traumatic experiences they encountered, managing and changing behaviour, supporting the education and development of the child, stopping the child from being in immediate risk or significant harm and improving their circumstances.

Direct work

In a recent publication examining the literature on effective interventions for children who have experience physical abuse, Montgomery and colleagues (2009) acknowledge that there is limited research on child-focused therapies, particularly those that involve only the child in treatment, although many different interventions exist. The researchers report that there is some evidence that individual child-parent focused intervention is effective, such as cognitive behaviour therapy, but that it is the parent component that may be the more effective element of such an intervention. The report continues that where the child is placed in care, treatment foster care interventions seem to be most promising for improving outcomes for children who have experienced maltreatment.

However, in a five year follow-up study on the outcomes for neglected children who had been returned home to families, Farmer and Lutman (2010) found that children who had experienced the most severe neglect had the poorest outcomes. The authors also found that children, who were older (mean 10.2 years) when returned home, had the poorest outcomes in terms of their well-being and stability in the family home; children with a mean age of 5.5 years when returned home had the best well-being. The researchers identified some children who had experienced abuse and/or neglect over long periods before a child protection plan was made. The length of time varied by local authority; the authors suggest that the threshold for children being made subject of a plan was too high in some authorities (see Box 5.2 for more information). This raises the concerning implication that the children for whom the outcomes are likely to be poorest are responded to the slowest.

Box 5.2 Research highlight

Farmer, E. and Lutman, E. (2010) *Case Management and Outcomes for Neglected Children Returned to their Parents: A Five Year Follow-Up Study (Research Brief).* London: Department for Education.

Farmer and Lutman studied a cohort of 138 neglected children from 104 families across seven local authorities who had been removed from home and then returned to their parents. The majority of the children had been included in a previous reunification study and the cohort had been followed for five years. Case files were reviewed and social workers, team managers and leaving care workers were interviewed about 50 of the children in more depth. Six parents and six children were also interviewed. All the children had been seriously neglected, but 65 per cent had also experienced emotional abuse, 61 per cent physical abuse and 27 per cent sexual abuse.

In a fifth of cases little or no support was offered. Parents of older children received less support than parents of younger children, although older children received more types of help than younger children. Overall the parents and children could have benefitted from more intensive support. Lack of specialist help was associated with poorer outcomes for children. After return home further referrals for about 73 per cent of the children were received and often insufficient action was taken in response.

In half of the cases there was inadequate attention to key issues and in many cases parental issues such as substance misuse, domestic abuse, mental health problems and lack of parenting skills were not tackled. Assessments had often not been undertaken and there was a lack of knowledge of the family history and key events. In particular, there were huge gaps in services for parental substance misuse. The authors suggest that parents need to be given clear messages that substance misuse will be monitored and reviewed 'before and during return'.

By the end of the five year period 43 per cent were living stably at home, 29 per cent were permanently adopted and 28 per cent had unstable experiences characterized by a mix of care and returns. The children living stably away from home were the most likely to be experiencing good well-being (although the figure was only 58%) while 70 per cent of those in unstable settings had poor outcomes. Living stably at home was not necessarily associated with good well-being outcomes, there was a spread with a third experiencing poor outcomes. Those in unstable situations were the oldest and those in the stable away from home settings were the youngest:

> ...children who were *under the age of six* at return were most likely to find stability in an alternative placement if the study return was not successful. For children who returned home *over the age of six* there was a heightened risk of having a subsequent unstable placement outcome, much less chance of ever achieving permanence in care and their cases were less well managed. The majority of children who were over 12 at return had unstable outcomes. (p.4)

The authors identified four patterns of case management.

1. 'Proactive' case management occurred in 25 per cent of cases. In these cases social care services responded to concerns about children and acted to protect them and make plans for the future. Parents were given the opportunity to demonstrate that they could care for their children, but action was taken if they were not able to and there was effective use of care proceedings and child

protection plans. This type of case management was associated with stability for children either away from home or back at home.

2. In 25 per cent of cases management was 'initially proactive but later became passive' and was characterized by prompt and effective early action, but a tailing off as time went by.

3. 26 per cent of cases were 'passively managed initially but management later became proactive', in others words, they were treated as 'family support' cases for too long despite indications of concern.

4. In 24 per cent of cases management was 'passive throughout' and children experienced long periods of harm that was not ameliorated. The cases were treated as 'family support', but little clear support was provided to tackle the presenting parenting issues. (p.3)

Overall, there were big variations between authorities in quality of practice and these variations were associated with variations in outcomes for children.

Children exposed to neglect may develop apathy, passivity and withdrawal along with behaviour problems and academic delay (Macdonald 2005). Therefore interventions that specifically address these difficulties need to be considered. While there is evidence of what works in improving children's emotional health or well-being (see, for example, McAuley, Pecora and Rose 2006), such interventions are likely to contribute to improved outcomes for neglected children, but do not necessarily focus on ameliorating the specific impact that neglect may have upon a child. A handful of studies from the US indicate that there may be a role for the involvement of peers as a means of reducing signs of withdrawal and increasing positive interaction and play among maltreated children, including those who have been neglected.

A review by Daro (1988) indicates that enhanced provision of services such as play therapy, additional education support, and speech and language therapy can greatly improve the functioning of abused or neglected children; although there is insufficient evidence on their effectiveness in terms of outcomes (Montgomery *et al.* 2009). However, provision of compensatory experiences and targeted support services for neglected children is important in order to promote a healthy developmental trajectory, and drawings may provide a means of communication for very young preschool children who may not be able to articulate their feelings clearly (Carpenter *et al.* 1997). See Box 5.3 for a case example.

Box 5.3 Case study

Aiden is 8 years old and living with his mother. Following a referral to a project providing support for previous domestic abuse, other issues emerged: mother's mental health, concerns about possible poverty as the family had little money to buy food. The family were living in temporary accommodation, consisting of one hotel room. After speaking with Aiden, it appeared that his mother had also hit him a few times. Aiden also was showing some aggressive behaviour including one incident where he had threatened his mother with a knife. The family were referred to social services under child protection procedures and also for mental health assessments.

The initial intervention offered included immediate provision of food. The provision of art therapy sessions allowed the worker to gain an understanding of Aiden's inner world, and they drew a series of very concerning conclusions, indicating the effects of emotional neglect, which helped to inform an assessment of his needs. The provision of art therapy for Aiden alongside emotional and practical support for his mother is a good example of multifaceted intervention in action. In this case, Aiden's mother's mental health assessment and the assessment of Aiden provided the gateway for further, targeted support services. Following his assessment, Aiden received a diagnosis of oppositional defiant disorder. Staff at the project ensured that Aiden was enabled to go on several day trips with other children, during which time his mother was provided with some counselling. This also gave his mother some much needed respite from her caring duties.

Another intervention used imaginative play training for emotionally neglected children in group sessions over five weeks. When evaluated in a randomized controlled trial, children receiving the intervention developed increased levels of imagination, cooperation with peers and used less aggressive play than the control group participants (Udwin 1983). Further evaluations of interventions for children are required before we can draw conclusions about what works.

Resilience-based approaches are increasingly used in direct work with children and a number of intervention strategies have been suggested (Benard 2004; Daniel and Wassell 2002; Luthar 2005; Masten 1994; Newman 2004; Rutter 1987). There is much to suggest that neglected children in particular could have a lot to gain from resilience-based approaches because the experience of neglect erodes the key factors associated with resilience. Neglect can affect the development of secure attachments, undermines self-esteem and impedes a sense of self-efficacy – all features of resilience. Intervention aimed at nurturing factors associated with resilience should help to reduce some of the worst outcomes of neglect over the longer term. However, research on the implementation of resilience-based approaches suggested that the term is often used loosely to denote a whole range of interventions that can broadly be defined as positive and solution-focused (Daniel *et al.* 2009). There can also be confusions about the intended outcomes and the routes to those outcomes. For example, one practitioner may say that they are boosting a child's self-esteem in order to improve their friendships while another may say that they are improving peer relationships in order to boost self-esteem. Where there is a network of practitioners involved they may not have a clear agreement about what the intended aims are nor how they should best attain those aims. This reiterates the importance of very clear and focused planning where the goals are set out clearly and the routes to those goals are defined (see Box 5.4).

Box 5.4 Activity

Research into factors associated with resilience has led to the development of a number of guiding frameworks for intervention via a range of protective factors. Rutter's framework (1987) suggests that practice should:

- alter or reduce the child's exposure to risk
- reduce the negative chain reaction of risk exposure
- establish and maintain self-esteem and self-efficacy
- create opportunities.

Masten's framework (1994) suggests that practitioners should aim to:

- reduce vulnerability and risk
- reduce the number of stressors and pile-up
- increase the available resources
- foster resilience strings
- alter or reduce the child's exposure to risk.

And Benard (2004) suggests the need for the child to experience:

- caring relationships
- high expectations
- opportunities to participate and contribute.

It is also important, as Luthar (2005) points out, to focus on factors that are 'modifiable modifiers', that is, they can be changed rather than being relatively fixed, as is, for example, gender.

Factors associated with resilience can be located at the level of the child, the family and the wider environment, and therefore, intervention by the protective network of practitioners should aim to address each of these layers of influence.

1. Think about a neglected child who is in need of support.

2. Consider the extent to which there has been an assessment of the three building blocks of resilience and if not, can you gauge levels of:

   a. secure attachment

   b. good self-esteem

   c. a sense of self-efficacy.

3. Consider whether there are opportunities to nurture resilience by considering six domains of the child's life:

   a. secure base

   b. education

   c. friendships

   d. talents and interests

   e. positive values

   f. social competencies. (Daniel and Wassell 2002)

4. Map out the intended outcomes and the proposed route to each outcome, it may help to draw a diagram.

5. Note which discipline's expertise will be needed to ensure a holistic response to the child and note which professional or para-professional within the helping network would be best placed to approach which task.

6. Note what will be needed to ensure that all involved are working towards the same goals and how progress will be monitored.

School-based support

The potential role of schools and teachers in providing therapeutic support for children is vast. The opportunity to learn in a stimulating environment with empathic staff can in itself be a protective factor that may reduce risks to neglected children. However, their peers may reject children who are neglected if they appear unkempt, smelly or dirty, and lack appropriate social skills. School can therefore be both an important arena for intervention as well as a source of feelings of shame and isolation for neglected children.

In many countries there are initiatives involving multi-disciplinary approaches, for example, basing social workers within schools. One such initiative in New Zealand – the Social Workers in Schools (SWIS) programme has been evaluated and shows much promise (Belgrave *et al.* 2002). The social workers use a strengths-based approach to respond flexibly to the needs of children and their families who can use the service on a voluntary basis. In addition to enhancing educational performance and improving behaviour in school, the intervention appeared to

> significantly improve circumstances for children who, at the beginning of the intervention, came to school hungry, not well clothed and whose health and hygiene were creating issues in classrooms and playgrounds. (p.9)

The evaluation also found increased use of clear family routines regarding food and bedtimes, and increased use of more positive communication strategies between parents and children. The voluntary nature of participation and the setting of social work intervention within a school rather than a statutory context enabled strong and effective relationships to be built with children and families.

Treatment foster care

An example of treatment foster care is the 'Multidimensional Treatment Foster Care' (National Implementation Team in England 2010) programme, which aims to develop effective placements and services for young people with complex welfare needs who are looked after by local authorities. Complex needs include offending, anti-social behaviour and severe emotional and behavioural difficulties. Programmes consist of training in behaviour management and positive parent–child interactions for the foster parents before receiving the child, daily telephone support and supervision, weekly group meetings, and 24-hour on-call crisis interventions. Alternatively, the New Orleans Intervention Model developed in Louisiana focuses on providing an intensive attachment-based programme of assessment and targeted interventions. Every child for whom there has been a court adjudication that maltreatment has occurred (and this is usually neglect) has a detailed assessment of each attachment relationship; and interventions are offered where appropriate (Zeanah *et al.* 2001). Where significant relationship change with the birth family has been achieved, children are rehabilitated back to the birth family. If not, a recommendation is made to the courts that the child should be freed for adoption. The attachment assessments and outcomes of any interventions feed in to this decision.

An evaluation of the four years prior to, compared with the four years since the introduction of the model has shown an increase in freeing for adoption. Moreover, for those children who do go back to their birth families, there is a significant reduction in maltreatment both for those children and for subsequent siblings (Zeanah *et al.* 2001). A seven year follow-up of 80 children exposed to the intervention has shown that on virtually all mental health measures, graduates of the New Orleans Intervention, whether adopted or rehabilitated, are similar to the general population. While further testing is required in different populations, the results are certainly promising.

Parent-focused interventions

Parent-focused interventions are directed at changing some aspect of a parent's well-being and to enable and support parents in caring for their children, or specific issues that hinder the parent's ability to care for their child or children. Research has identified a number of types of approach that had been evaluated in terms of their effectiveness – cognitive behavioural programmes; psychotherapeutic interventions, and home visiting programmes.

There are certain parental difficulties that are thought to be particularly likely to give rise to neglect of children. Such circumstances include families in which parents are misusing substances and also families in which parents are experiencing mental health problems, including maternal depression. However, we need to bear in mind that a diagnosis of parental substance abuse or dependence, depression or other mental health problem does not necessarily mean that a child is at risk. Parental behaviour and children's needs should be considered regardless of the label that may have been applied to them (Duncan and Reder 2000; Velleman and Orford 1999). The impact on children may not be the same in every case, even within the same family, due to each child's individual characteristics and their personal strengths and vulnerabilities or family circumstances. Again, individual parental risk behaviours and individual children's needs have to be considered in each case (Moran 2009). However, parents of older children often receive significantly less support than those with younger children, even when the older children receive more types of help than younger ones. Lack of specialist help for parents has been linked to poorer outcomes for children (Farmer and Lutman 2010). In many cases Farmer and Lutman found that children were returned home without the problems that affected parenting in the first place having been addressed.

Parent education and support

Among the many parent education and training programmes that have been developed over the past two decades, there have been few that have specifically been designed to tackle neglect. However, one programme that has been well evaluated and tackles many of the factors associated with neglect is a programme from the US called Project 12 Ways. It earns its name from the twelve core services that comprised the original intervention: parent–child training, stress reduction for parents, basic skill training for children, money management training, social support, home safety training, multiple-setting behaviour management in situ, health and nutrition, problem-solving, couples counselling, alcohol abuse referral, and single mother services. Studies indicate that the programme leads to a reduction in child abuse and neglect but its impact may not be sustained long-term (Macdonald 2001). It is possible that 'booster services' may be required or other forms of additional support for families to maintain the gains acquired from the programme (Macdonald 2005).

Another example is a group-based parent-training form of cognitive behavioural therapy known as Triple-P (Sanders *et al.* 2004). The evidence suggests that the use of Triple-P (Positive Parenting Programme) improves the parenting of young children (aged 2 to 7 years) by parents some of whom had been referred to a child protection authority for potential abuse or neglect and/or parents having difficulty expressing their anger (Barlow and Schrader-MacMillan 2009). See Box 5.5 for a case example.

Box 5.5 Case study

Mrs Taylor was referred to children's services. She was a single mother to three children under the age of ten, and suffered from depression and chronic back pain. The family's living conditions were damp and unhygienic, and the school were concerned about the children's appearance and personal hygiene. There was concern that Mrs Taylor was unable to pick up on the children's expressed needs and behavioural cues. Supports were put in place to address mental health issues, family routines in the home, and speech and language therapy for the children, and Mrs Taylor was referred to the Triple-P programme.

The application of a structured programme allowed Mrs Taylor to focus on her parenting and how it impacted on her children's daily life. For example, Mrs Taylor's ability to manage her youngest child's tantrums improved significantly as a result of her learning and support within the Triple-P programme. Mrs Taylor ceased her overuse of a permissive discipline style and was able to manage routines and boundaries better in the home, and improve the daily life of her children; the application of parenting skills learned within the Triple-P course meant that her son was able to successfully sit and enjoy a mealtime routine.

The Triple-P programme was a key element in the range of interventions that were organized to support Mrs Taylor and her family. Triple-P offered the teaching of skills to the mother and a structured way of measuring outcomes in her application of them, allowing for meaningful change to take place.

Parental substance misuse

Around one in five families referred to children's social services in the UK have a history of alcohol or drugs problems (Cleaver *et al.* 1999), rising to one in two families on the Child Protection Register (Forrester 2000), and affecting three out of four families involved in care proceedings (Hayden and Johnson 2000).

Parental substance misuse (including either drugs or alcohol) may impact on children in a number of ways. Barnard and Barlow (2003) report that children's discovery of their parents' substance misuse is associated with feelings of hurt, rejection, anger, sadness, and anxiety about the well-being of the parent. Children describe their parents who misuse substances as moody, sleepy, spending little time with them, and never having any money to spend. Sometimes there is concern about role reversal and caring responsibilities being placed on the shoulders of children, and concerns about them having missed out on childhood opportunities for play and learning, although, as noted in Chapter 3, it is important not to make assumptions or use terms such as 'parentification' without careful assessment of the child's experience.

Robust studies of evaluations that provide evidence of what works are a handful based in the US programmes. The best known and most thoroughly evaluated is 'Strengthening Families' which was devised for parents who misuse substances and their 3 to 17 year old children. The programme was designed in order to reduce family environmental risk factors and enhance protective factors, hence increasing personal resilience and fostering resistance to substance misuse. Its focus is on family environments, and specifically on helping parents develop their parenting skills (Kumpfer and Tait 2000).

Parental mental health

Symptoms of depression including hopelessness, low self-worth and poor concentration may reduce parents' emotional availability to a child, thus impacting on children's attachment security and own sense of self-worth. These effects can be particularly damaging when children are very young and hence the need for early detection of difficulties via, for example, peri- and post-natal screening for depression in mothers. Treatment needs to be tailored to support parents' specific needs such as psychotherapy for depression and anxiety, including cognitive behavioural therapy (Austin and Priest 2004) or social network building to overcome isolation.

Evidence regarding what works in cases of parents who are depressed and whose children are neglected is minimal, with studies more often reporting on parenting programmes for mothers with depression focusing on reduction of children's conduct problems as an outcome rather than on measures of neglect. One exception is a Jamaican study of home visiting for undernourished children (age 9 months to 30 months) and their mothers with depression (Baker-Henningham *et al.* 2005). The families in the study received weekly home visits by community health aides for one year, who showed mothers how to play with their child using home-made materials, and discussed parenting issues. Mothers who received at least 25 visits over the year reported a significant reduction in depression symptoms, and reduced maternal depression was associated with improved children's development, but only for boys.

Domestic abuse

The third parental factor associated with child neglect, domestic abuse is highly damaging for children. Moreover, domestic abuse tends to a co-morbidity with mental health issues and substance misuse and disaggregation of the three can be tricky. Interventions have generally been targeted at the adult: either as perpetrators or as victims – and some have been fairly successful. However, even those that are not direct perpetrator programmes and address parenting attitudes and behaviours, such as the Canadian originated 'Caring Dads' (Scott 2008; Scott and Crooks 2004), do not capture routine data about the impact on children. A recent innovation from the NSPCC has added a children's element to this programme and is currently under evaluation (Taylor 2010).

For children living with domestic abuse however, what seems to work best are interventions that target reparation of the relationship between the child and the non-abusing parent. It is common for mothers and children not to talk to each other about the abuse. This silence makes it very difficult for children to express their feelings. Quite often a mother may not fully realize how aware her children are of the violence and how it affects them. Mothers who have suffered domestic violence need reassurance that there is a 'legacy of secrecy' and a pattern of protecting one another from painful knowledge. These may be difficult patterns to break (Hester, Pearson and Harwin 2007; Mullender *et al.* 2002).

Exciting research by Humphreys *et al.* (2006) has shown promise in working with mothers and children in parallel to explore these relationships. The CEDAR programme (Children Experiencing Domestic Abuse Recovery) is currently under review, but is showing promise in working with that relationship (Violence Against Women Scotland 2009). The NSPCC are currently delivering and testing a similar model called DART (Domestic Abuse: Recovering Together) that uses groupwork with mothers and children together throughout the programme. Early results of all are promising: what seems key is that focusing on mother–child relationship appears most helpful.

Parent–child focused interventions

Parent- and child-focused interventions are explicitly directed at changing aspects of parent–child interactions that are thought to contribute to emotionally abusive interactions. The literature identified two key theoretical approaches underpinning parent-and child-focused interventions – psychotherapeutic and attachment-based models (Barlow and Schrader-MacMillan 2009).

Preschool parent psychotherapy

Preschool parent psychotherapy (PPP) addresses the relationship between mother and child by focusing on and making links between the mother's history and responses to her child. The limited evidence suggests that this method of working with emotionally abusive parents was effective in reducing children's difficult interactions with mothers, and actually led to a greater improvement in what each expected from the relationship (Barlow and Schrader-MacMillan 2009).

Video Interaction Guidance (VIG)

VIG is primarily focused on training caregivers to respond sensitively to their infants, by using brief clips of the parent and infant interacting, to highlight and demonstrate sensitive interaction and its benefits. One of the important aspects of VIG is focusing on any examples of positive interaction, pointing these out to the parent and encouraging them to do more of the same. It can be a powerful tool because it can often be difficult for practitioners to articulate exactly what needs to be different. Being able to point out what is required on screen can, therefore, be very effective. Parents can also be encouraged to observe the child's reaction. For example, if eye contact is made, even briefly, with the child, there can be a strong positive reaction from the child.

Limited findings suggest as a result of VIG mothers can show improvements in maternal sensitivity, and a significant decrease in the level of disrupted communication (see Macdonald and Lugton 2006).

Family-focused interventions

Family-focused interventions are directed at the whole family, and are aimed at improving interaction and relationships between family members, and supporting the family's self-sufficiency, inclusion in society and general well-being.

In spite of the attention given to the contribution of family therapy and family systems theory, there are few quantitative studies on the effectiveness of family-focused interventions. Family therapy or family preservation services have not, to date, shown promising outcomes, and the stronger evidence for these interventions in the form of randomized trials report mixed results. The effectiveness of family therapy is unclear given that one randomized trial compared it with CBT, showing family therapy to be equally or less effective (Barlow and Schrader-MacMillan 2009; Montgomery *et al.* 2009).

Following on from the success of the Head Start programme in the US, the UK government launched Sure Start in 1998. It is a community-wide initiative aimed at preventing the social exclusion of disadvantaged children, from conception to age fourteen years (and older for those with special education needs). Sure Start aims to promote physical, emotional, intellectual and social development in preschool children by increasing childcare availability, supporting parents in employment and in developing their careers, providing parent skills training and education on child development, health and family support services. Although not specifically designed to tackle neglect, this initiative addresses several of the factors that are thought to contribute to neglect.

A large-scale, six-year evaluation of all Sure Start programmes in England, led by the Institute for the Study of Children, Families and Social Issues, University of London, initially showed a mixed picture regarding its effectiveness with less disadvantaged families benefitting more than the most disadvantaged (National Evaluation of Sure Start 2005). However, a later study (National Evaluation of Sure Start 2008) found beneficial effects for almost all children and families living in Sure Start areas. This was attributed to more effective outreach to the households requiring greater help. This report has paved the way for greater use of outreach and the move towards children's centres in England becoming centres for targeted rather than universal services. These findings reassert the need for practitioners to develop trusting relationships with parents and then provide the bridge to a range of services.

Home visiting

There are several home visiting programmes that are effective or at least show promise in tackling neglect. They typically involve a professional or trained person visiting vulnerable families with the aim of enhancing a number of factors such as child health and diet, maternal parenting skills, attachment, social support and involvement with services.

Barlow and Schrader-MacMillan (2009) identified a number of studies that evaluated the effectiveness of home visiting interventions with groups of parents in whom emotional maltreatment was of concern or there were severe difficulties in the parents' relationship with their child. One interesting study examined the benefits for parents of infants defined as having non-organic failure to thrive (faltering growth) of combining 'lay' home visitors (home visitors supervised by a community health nurse) aimed at providing support to the mother and promoting parenting, and the child's development (Black *et al.* 2007). The intervention was delivered during one year and was compared with services provided through clinics only. The results showed that lay home visitors contributed to the improvement of language development in young children, better home environment for the child, and improved cognition in younger children. The children were followed-up at aged 8 and the findings showed that home visiting had helped to reduce some of the effects of early failure to thrive, possibly by promoting the mother's sensitivity to the child and helping children to benefit more from school.

Overall, the results of these evaluations are conflicting with regard to the benefits of home visiting and this reflects the diversity in the nature of the home visiting programmes evaluated, the limited populations with whom they have been evaluated (e.g. drug abusing and faltering growth), and the different outcomes used.

Social network interventions

A characteristic of families where children are neglected is their social isolation. Social network interventions aim to extend and strengthen social support available to such families. A study by Gaudin (1993a) indicates that it is possible to reduce the likelihood of neglect in families when their social support networks are bolstered in this way. The specific project reported by Gaudin involved families undergoing a comprehensive assessment to identify the problems they faced, the size and quality of their supportive network, and the difficulties in accessing support (such as lack of a telephone, poor social skills or low self-esteem). The intervention itself involved use of five specific social network interventions in combination with professional case work/management, including advocacy and brokering of formal services. The social network interventions took a number of forms, some of which overlap with components of programmes described above:

- *Personal networking* – involving direct intervention to enhance existing relationships and potential relationships with family, relatives, neighbours or work associates.

- *Establishing mutual aid groups* – aiming to teach parenting and social skills, and develop problem-solving ability and enhance self-esteem.

- *Volunteer linking* – involving use of trained volunteers to carry out tasks similar to family aides.

- *Recruiting neighbours as informal helps* – who are paid a small amount and receive support and guidance from social workers.

- *Social skills training* – aimed at overcoming skills deficits that may interfere with the formation of supportive relationships.

More than three quarters of the parents who received this intervention for at least nine months improved their parenting from neglectful or severely neglectful to marginally adequate parenting according to a standardized measure. However, there was a high dropout rate, and families participated on a voluntary basis and similar results might not be achieved with families who are more reluctant to receive help or do not see what it may offer them (Moran 2007).

Therapeutic interventions

Therapeutic interventions with families in cases of neglect are more likely to be successful if they are inclusive of extra-familial factors that influence family functioning (Macdonald 2005). Multi-systemic family therapy (MST) is an approach that involves a combination of intervention strategies aimed at addressing risk and protective factors at individual, family and social levels. It combines strategic family therapy, structural family therapy and cognitive behaviour therapy, and involves families working intensively with a dedicated therapist. Although this approach has mostly been used to work with violent or criminal young people and their families, it has also been used with families where there is neglect or abuse. It has been found to reduce parental stress, social isolation, and improve parent–child relationships including parental responsiveness (Brunk, Henggeler and Whelan 1987). However, in terms of working with families where children are neglected, this approach can only be described currently as promising, as direct measures of child abuse or neglect were not assessed, and there has been no long-term follow-up (Macdonald 2005).

Conclusions

Neglect is an umbrella term that covers numerous different issues and, importantly, it can affect children of any age. Studies into effective interventions to reduce the impact and reoccurrence of neglect are few in number. However, we can identify common factors about effective interventions.

The evidence points to the need for intensive multilevel interventions or methods of working that target not only parenting practices, but factors that may be operating within the parent(s) including mental health problems, partner violence, and parental alcohol and drugs problems. Support is needed to help parents' manage their children's behaviour, parenting skills and domestic violence (Barlow and Schrader-MacMillan 2009, Farmer and Lutman 2010). For children who have been looked after, greater clarity with parents about what changes need to be made, over what timescales before children are returned to them, together with intensive packages of assistance are required (Farmer and Lutman 2010).

The overall conclusion is that practitioners need to plan intervention very carefully to address each of the issues identified for children and parents. They also need to consider the nature of engagement, the quality of the working relationship and the views of parents and children about what would help them most.

KEY MESSAGES

1. Interventions need to offer long-term support for families where there are difficulties in order that the benefits of short-term and focused interventions can be sustained.

2. Interventions need to be multifaceted and deal with all aspects of neglect, both personal and practical in order to treat the whole 'system'. Close working and analysis of service effectiveness with practitioners across all agencies is needed to turn this into reality and thus avoid 'drift'.

3. The provision of a supportive yet challenging relationship to a parent and/or child or young person is critical to enable individuals to have the confidence to face issues and make the changes. Support offered outside such a relationship is likely to be experienced by family members as demanding or instructive and while there are cases where this approach is necessary, it is an approach less likely to reduce neglect within the family.

4. Activities towards improving the self-esteem of children, young people and parents and carers are highlighted as a feature of effective interventions. Achievement can strengthen resilience for vulnerable families and this resilience can in turn provide confidence to parent in improved ways and to deal more effectively with some of the omissions of care.

5. Interventions should include all key people in the child's life and particular care must be taken not to ignore male figures whether present in or absent from the home. Any risks they may pose should be considered along with any positive aspects they may bring to the care of the child.

6. Direct work with children is often neglected, but in the long run may have the most beneficial effects – especially in situations where parents' problems are seriously entrenched.

7. Working in partnership with schools to provide support for children's emotional, cognitive and behavioural development is essential.

School-based support can be linked with wider class-room initiatives aimed at building self-esteem and self-efficacy.

8. Intervention aimed at tackling the core issues leading to the concern in the first place is essential. If there are factors that are known to be affecting parenting, such as substance misuse, mental health issues or domestic abuse then they must be directly targeted.

9. Intervention that aims to improve the relationship between the child and parent/s can improve attachment relationships and the parent's attunement to the child's needs.

10. Neglected children need the expertise of all key disciplines and no one profession is likely to be able to provide all the support that children need to flourish. Therefore, the expertise and resources of all should be pooled so that the resulting whole is greater than the sum of the parts.

6

Preventing Child Neglect

Introduction

Our review of the literature suggested that the current UK policy initiatives are, in the main, congruent with the emergent evidence base about children's developmental needs and the proximal and distal factors that affect parenting capacity. The review also suggested that many professionals have the knowledge and skills required to respond to children who may be neglected. The area about which there is less evidence is how public and voluntary services can best ensure that children's developmental needs are met, whatever the level of parental capacity.

The biggest gap in evidence we identified related to the views of parents and, even more, of children about what kind of services they would access and the supports required to bridge the gap between the capacity to articulate anxieties and to act on them. The term 'hard to reach' is often used to denote parents who exhibit the kind of characteristics associated with neglect, however, we suggest that services should actively seek more evidence about what it is that makes them 'hard to access' for some people.

We wanted to draw the book to a positive conclusion by suggesting ways that child neglect might be prevented. Our argument is simply this: public health approaches have the potential to make a significant difference to the way we approach child protection, not only as a useful metaphor, but as an emergent method on which we advocate further work (Scott and Taylor 2010).

The landscape of child protection

The landscape of child protection has changed and we are probably now at the edge of a third wave (Scott 2009):

- In the first wave (late 19th century), the plight of destitute and neglected children was recognized (e.g. NSPCC) and there was an increased role in loco parentis, as well as significant involvement by the church.

- During the second wave (mid-late 20th century), there was the uncovering of hidden problems of physical and sexual abuse, which led to an emphasis on 'identify and notify' within policy and the increased role of the state in child protection. This is now fraught with demand pressures; difficulties in assessment; and a multiplicity of co-existent problems.

- The early 21st century heralds the emergence of opportunities for prevention based on a greater understanding of child maltreatment and closely related problems.

It seems to us that a public health approach affords the greatest prospects in dealing with this third wave, where we are beginning to accumulate an evidence base of preventive activities in neglect; where we know so much more about the antecedents and consequences of neglect than we ever did before. Early intervention has become something of a mantra, but nowhere is it more crucial than in neglect – early in the life cycle, early recognition, early response after detection. These three 'early' principles are absolutely key in preventing neglect.

The costs of neglect

There are some very convincing reasons for an approach to child protection that is based on an ecological model and that focuses attention on both decreasing risk factors and bolstering protective and resilience factors. The consequences of child maltreatment are serious and significant: for the individual, for society as a whole, and potentially for future generations. The costs, both direct (e.g. medical care) and indirect (e.g. criminal justice, education, specialist provision) of addressing these consequences are enormous (Browne, Hamilton-Giachritis and Vettor 2007). In Europe only the UK has attempted to calculate the total economic burden of maltreatment – in 1996 this was estimated as £735 million (Mostyn 1996). Garrison (2005) argues that we know enough about child maltreatment to have an impact, but we lack the political will. She suggests that we need to persuade electorates and governments that we can afford preventive and treatment measures, and convince them that we cannot afford the current high rates of abuse and neglect. See also McIntosh *et al.*'s study (2009) highlighted in Box 6.1.

Box 6.1 Research highlight

McIntosh, E., Barlow, J., Davis, H. and Stewart-Brown, S. (2009) 'Economic evaluation of an intensive home visiting programme for vulnerable families: A cost-effectiveness analysis of a public health intervention.' *Journal of Public Health, 31*, 423–433.

Home visiting programmes targeting vulnerable families to address parenting practices have the potential to improve long-term outcomes for children. Economic evaluations of these are rarely carried out however. McIntosh *et al.* (2009) undertook the first economic evaluation alongside a randomized controlled trial (RCT) on intensive home visiting.

One hundred and thirty-one women were identified as 'at risk' of abusing and neglecting their children by community midwives during the antenatal period. The at risk criteria included (among other things): being under age 17; serious housing problems; significant financial difficulties; psychiatric history; history of drug or alcohol problems; a previous child registered with child protective services. The women were randomly allocated to services as usual, or to an intensive home visiting programme. The intervention, lasting 18 months, comprised intensive weekly home visits from a trained home visitor working in partnership with the parents using the Family Partnership Project. The unit costs of each stage of both the intervention arm and care as usual were calculated using sophisticated economic measures.

The home visiting programme improved maternal sensitivity and better enabled home visitors to identify infants in need of further protection at an incremental cost of £3246 per woman. While home visiting interventions are always more costly, the effects for the infant are almost always more effective. However, it depends on how much value is placed on outcomes such as maternal sensitivity.

The research was funded by the Department of Health and the Nuffield Foundation.

The consequences of neglect

The consequences of neglect are generally cumulative and often negatively affect the child's development. Neglect often accompanies other forms of abuse, but is the one that is most overlooked. Box 6.2 highlights a research study by Anda and Felitti (2010) on this theme.

Box 6.2 Research highlight

Anda, R. and Felitti, V. (2010) 'The Adverse Childhood Experiences (ACE) Study [online].' Available at www.acestudy.org/, accessed on 2 June 2010.

There is undeniable evidence of the long-term damage and effects of childhood neglect and abuse from the Adverse Childhood Events series. During the 1980s and early 1990s information about risk factors for disease had been widely researched and merged into public education and prevention programmes. However, it was also clear that a number of these common disease risk factors (such as smoking, misusing alcohol, sexual behaviours, physical inactivity, etc.) were not randomly distributed in the population. Moreover, risk factors for many chronic diseases seem to cluster together. In other words, individuals with one risk factor tend also to have one or more others.

This was useful knowledge, but left lots of gaps about what the origins might be regarding those risk factors. The ACE Study was designed to work out what might be the linkages between Adverse Childhood Experiences (or ACEs) and risk factors that lead to poor health and social consequences. Specifically, the ACE study is beginning to provide data that will help answer the question: 'If risk factors for disease, disability, and early mortality are not randomly distributed, what influences precede the adoption or development of them?' In doing so, it is possible that new prevention programmes and interventions might be designed.

To date there have been 18,000 participants and over 50 academic publications from the study. The conceptual framework clearly demonstrates the whole-life approach and how risk factors derived from adverse childhood experiences can accumulate. The ACE study does not currently differentiate between abuse and neglect, but what is very clear is that childhood maltreatment has long-term health effects. In comparison to the general population, adults who were harmed as children are 103 per cent more likely to smoke; 43 per cent more likely to become suicidal; 103 per cent more likely to become alcohol dependent; and 192 per cent more likely to develop addiction to drugs. And they are also more likely to become teenage parents, develop mental health problems, be obese; develop diabetes, cardiovascular disease, etc; use more health and social care resources.

Why we suggest a public health approach to neglect

A public health approach directly addresses the call to move away from traditional responses that aim to prevent recurrence of maltreatment to preventing it happening at all (Daro and Dodge 2009; Stagner and Lansing 2009), while simultaneously acknowledging the importance of a full spectrum of action that might require a differential response. A public health approach to child protection can do this, although the language may be unfamiliar to some. A public health approach may be best understood as something slightly more than a metaphor, albeit not quite yet a method in child protection (Scott and Taylor 2010). There are three particular reasons why we would advocate a public health approach (Scott 2009):

1. The prevalence and the long-term effects of child abuse are so utterly serious (Gilbert *et al.* 2009a; Gilbert *et al.* 2009b; MacMillan *et al.* 2009; Reading *et al.* 2009). In neglect, these are perhaps the most severe, not least because neglected children remain under the radar of professional awareness for too long, and outside the circle of protective intervention until far too late. Child neglect constitutes by far the majority of cases of significant harm to children (Gardner 2010). And while some forms of abuse are clearly decreasing, emotional abuse has increased (Barlow 2008).

2. The current 'cure' of removing children from homes where they are being maltreated is harming many children (Doyle 2007; Rubin *et al.* 2007). Not only might such an intervention occur too late, the subsequent breakdown of placements, the shuttling to and fro between foster care and reunification and the length of time to find permanent placements is for many children absolutely bleak. There are around 83,000 children in care at any one time in the UK alone, a further 2000 in secure youth service settings (Hendry 2010). By the time children come into care they may have already suffered years of neglect and abuse. And the care system itself often harms them further, either by being too late to compensate for previous harm, or indeed by compounding that harm (Taylor 2010). After years of interventions, it seems we have made significantly little inroad into improving the situation (Garrison 2005).

3. Demand has far outstripped the capacity of child protection systems to respond effectively, evidenced in serious case reviews and their equivalents throughout the world. Gill's (2010) analysis of the events leading up to the death of Peter Connelly demonstrates starkly not only how many missed opportunities there were for an effective

response, but also issues of thresholds being set too high, lack of a coordinated overview and systemic demands on and flaws within the system. Unfortunately we know this is a picture repeated over and over.

So for these three very good reasons, evidenced throughout this book, intervening too little and too late is better than not intervening at all, but only just. The consequences of neglect for individual children are harsh and we have a moral obligation to respond effectively and early if we can. If we are not convinced by the moral case, then the economic and social cases are equally compelling. The costs to society and to the taxpayer are immense. Not just in dealing with children within the care system, but addressing the consequences: within education, the criminal justice system, the health service and so forth. If this was any other clinical problem on such a scale and with such devastating consequences we would have thrown enormous collective effort into addressing it. It is quite unbelievable that we have not done so for child neglect. Maltreatment is one of the biggest paediatric public-health challenges, yet any research activity is dwarfed by work on more established childhood ills (Horton 2003).

Misconceptions about public health

While we believe that public health approaches to child protection may be useful, it is acknowledged that the language is not always helpful and we have found that some child protection practitioners interpret this as suggesting a health needs and medically-led approach. Given that there are a number of misconceptions when using public health language, it is important to clarify what is *not* meant by a public health approach (Scott and Taylor 2010):

- it is not concerned only with responding to major epidemics
- it does not mean 'going soft' on abuse or neglect
- it does not make children responsible for behaviour change or prevention
- it is not solely about primary prevention or health promotion
- it does not mean it is a job only for health authorities or practitioners
- it does not mean we cannot act until we have complete understanding
- it is not a prescribed set of methods.

Rather, a public health approach is an overall framework within which to understand the delivery landscape. It is concerned with promoting well-being and curbing the ill-effects of social behaviours as much as it is about responding to outbreaks. The UK National Institute for Clinical Excellence (NICE) has recently generated a helpful schema on which to base public health guidance (Kelly *et al.* 2009), and key is the transaction across sectors:

> Positive and negative causal pathways cross physical, biological, social, economic, political and psychological discipline boundaries. (p.14)

The most common misconception is that a public health approach to child maltreatment is about health services – but it is not. Scott (2010) suggests we consider skin cancer as an example, where it is clear that strategies such as tackling the hole in the ozone layer are not about health services at all. Similarly the most important approaches to controlling infectious diseases are not about medical services, rather they are about sanitation and clean water. The range of possible interventions in relation to preventing child neglect is very broad. They thus need to be mapped out in relation to both risk and protective factors and within the context of specific opportunities to intervene early in the causal pathways (Scott and Taylor 2010).

A public health approach to neglect

It is implicit within the United Nations Convention on the Rights of the Child (United Nations 1989) that child maltreatment of all forms is preventable, and is thus not inevitable. The World Health Organization (WHO) suggests that methods to achieve this should be both systematic and multisectoral (Butchart, Harvey and Fumiss 2006). Such approaches are frequently encountered within the field of public health. While often referred to as a public health model, they are used in a multiplicity of fields. The WHO report (Butchart *et al.* 2006) suggests within these approaches action is taken to:

- prevent the problem from occurring
- detect the problem and respond when it does occur
- minimize its long-term negative effects.

And thus within the realm of child protection this means:

- implementing measures to prevent violence to children
- detecting cases and intervening early

- providing ongoing care to victims and families where maltreatment occurs

- preventing the reoccurrence of abuse and neglect.

A public health approach to child protection then provides a framework that basically shifts the balance in a number of ways (Barlow 2008): emphasizing the causes of problems at a population level rather than an individual one; recognizing that behaviour changes need to be made universally; and moving further towards prevention.

Butchart *et al.* (2006) outline the crucial elements involved in such a systematic approach to child protection. Briefly, these elements comprise:

- *Definitions*: common conceptual and operation definitions to enable case enumeration and identification.

- *Prevention*: policies and programmes that address both risk and protective factors.

- *Services*: comprehensive responses.

- *Information for effective action*: strengthening of methods that gather data and make it widely available.

- *Advocacy*: efforts in awareness raising among decision-makers and the public of the need for evidence-based prevention programmes; and for campaigns that focus on non-violent social and cultural norms, especially those that relate to parenting.

The river of child neglect

Within a public health approach the life continuum is commonly presented as the metaphor of a river, adapted slightly here for a child protection scenario. Practitioners stand at a point downstream on the river bank and can watch children floating past, often flailing and really struggling, sometimes already dead, always harmed. We have become extremely good at rescuing children and families from this point in the river, we can even save some from drowning. Our resuscitation techniques and lifeboats and communication processes are now quite sophisticated. But by the time these children have reached this point in the river, they are far downstream and their survival mechanisms are already seriously compromised. So if we are really going to tackle the huge numbers and make better progress with successful recovery from being in this river, we need to look at why they were in the water in the first place. We need a strong contingent of people to also consider going up the river and checking out what is happening there, and targeting solid interventions upstream. Are children being pushed into the river, do they jump, or do they fall in accidentally? If we can stop them getting into the water at all, then we would need very little effort downstream and just a little bit more at midstream points. Thus efforts to increase effective rescue (more children saved) mean a shift from a focus on the causes of problems at an individual level to ones at a population level (see Figure 6.1)

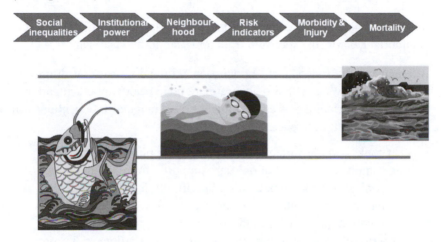

Figure 6.1: Illustrating the analogy of looking further upstream for the source of the problems identified downstream

Primary, secondary and tertiary interventions

Within a public health model for neglect, interventions are described as primary, secondary and tertiary. Primary protection interventions (upstream approaches) are preventive and apply to the entire population. The intention is to prevent child neglect before it occurs. Secondary prevention interventions (or midstream approaches) are focused on specific at risk populations or individuals, designed to target and prevent neglect from happening. Tertiary interventions (or downstream approaches) are therapeutic, aimed at minimizing further harm and promoting recovery.

Learning from public health interventions

We might argue that road trauma is a better example of a problem with many interrelated causes and the need for multiple strategies at each of these levels (Scott and Taylor 2010). Here too, great advances have been made by evidence-based strategies that include:

- safer car design
- better road engineering
- improved driver education
- new laws (e.g. seat belts, speeding fines, mobile phone use and drink driving penalties)
- law enforcement.

It is the combination of actions at primary, secondary and tertiary levels that is important, across the spectrum from upstream to downstream.

Alternatively, the Independent Enquiry on Scotland's misuse of drugs and alcohol (Matthews 2010) also advocates a public health approach and uses the decrease in smoking as an example where a range of interventions can make a significant difference:

> It took a whole variety of interventions applied with political commitment and bottom-up support from individuals, organizations and communities. Specifically it took smoke free policies, price regulation, public education, control of product promotion (advertising and sponsorship), proven treatments, control of package design and labelling, prosecutions, point of sale interventions and advocacy about tobacco and its industry. Smoking has declined because of a large number of synergistic interventions working together. In 2006, Scotland introduced a ban on smoking in public places. The press often treat this as an individual public health breakthrough but it is better seen as the last in a long line of interventions to reduce smoking and to protect others from passive smoking. (p.17)

Success is a non-event

At a population level it can be clear where a public health approach, using a range of interventions, has worked. Diseases once common may be eradicated (e.g. smallpox) or be brought under such control that they are on the verge of eradication (for instance polio). The problem of course is that sometimes it can also be very difficult to see if a public health approach really does make a difference. Swine flu sparked fears of an international pandemic during 2009 (the 'catch it, bin it, burn it' campaign). It caused 457 deaths in the UK in 2010 (Scottish Government 2010b), with numbers slightly down on 2009. People who worked in the health sector all felt the burden of responsibility. Plans were made throughout the health service for vaccination rosters and extra staff. Contingency plans for all projected scenarios were concocted. Universities and the health service worked in tandem to ensure student doctors and nurses (and those who taught them) could be deployed to help in less specialized clinical areas, freeing up more experienced staff to deal with the potential influx of critically ill patients, many of whom would be young children or very elderly and frail adults. Weekly teleconferences were held with senior representatives and the Chief Nursing Officer and representatives. Daily emails on the latest state of the H1N1 virus were beamed onto the computers of anyone who had a remote connection with the health service. There were simply numerous missives and updates, and all health sector researchers were implored to try and come up with solutions.

Then of course the expected pandemic did not happen and everyone was left wondering what the fuss was about and why we spent all that money. Instead of recognizing that it did not happen because we invested heavily upstream – extremely effectively.

It is unlikely that we are going to eradicate child neglect within the next generation or two. Dreadful cases are still going to come to our attention and will detract from efforts to shift upstream. We are never going to be able to know precisely how many children were not neglected because of our preventive methods, just like we do not know how many people did not get swine flu. We should not be distracted by that. A successful outcome in prevention is a non-event. Just like in skin cancer, smoking, road trauma and swine flu, it is not only those who were likely to suffer or die who are better off as a result. Going for a meal or drink now means clothes do not smell afterwards. But more importantly, as fewer people smoke, it is likely to mean significant savings on public expenditure for those whose health and well-being have been incapacitated by smoking-related diseases. The benefits should be equally as great in neglect.

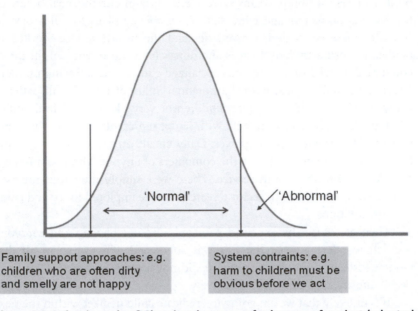

Figure 6.2: What is neglect? Showing the range of tolerance of neglect (adapted from Barlow 2008)

Barlow (2008) demonstrates graphically how this might work in practice, using physical abuse of children as an example, adapted here for neglect. Figure 6.2 is illustrative only, but shows how a diversity of views can be arranged. On the left hand side would be a view that suggests it is anathema to say that children can be dirty and smelly and happy. On the right would be a tolerance within society under system constraints that would expect children to be defined as neglected only once the consequences of neglect are clearly visible.

If a public health approach to neglect were then introduced, with a variety of universal strategies that took a population approach to tackling the problem, the whole balance would be shifted to the left (see Figure 6.3). A population-level approach would reduce the mean level of risk factors, and focus on a shift in societal norms. The result: a much narrower margin of children who fall through the neglect net.

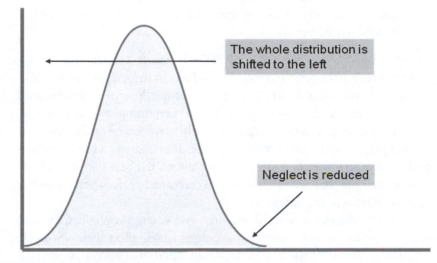

The whole distribution is shifted to the left

Neglect is reduced

Figure 6.3: Universal strategies: Showing the implications of taking a public health approach to neglect (adapted from Barlow 2008)

Applying the lessons

If we were to apply the lessons from a public health approach to problems like skin cancer and road trauma to the prevention of child neglect we would therefore (Scott and Taylor 2010):

1. Adopt a broad approach across different sectors and levels of government (e.g. health, education, social services).

2. Identify all known major risk and protective factors for child neglect and identify which risk factors can be reduced and which protective factors can be increased at a population level. We will need a range of interventions at different points of the river bank. Currently these are mainly focused downstream, we need to be shifting that balance of planning and priority further upstream.

3. Make a long-term commitment to these strategies – this means it needs to be a priority right across the political spectrum (and at state and federal levels in countries with such structures). Like the smoking ban, without state sponsored support and commitment it is going to be very hard to make a difference.

4. Base all strategies on high quality research on cost effectiveness otherwise there is a risk of causing further harm, and wasting scarce resources.

5. Be clear from the beginning what the benefits are to wider society and economy so that the exponential improvements in public life can be appreciated by all.

Getting it Right for Every Child (GIRFEC) (Scottish Government 2008) provides a useful blueprint and mechanism for a strategic approach to child welfare and protection. GIRFEC as it has become known is the national approach in Scotland to working with and supporting all children and young people. It is a public health approach based on research, evidence and best practice and works across all services for children and adults where children may be involved. It aims to give children the best start possible to improve their life chances, and involves all carers and professionals working together effectively and efficiently.

GIRFEC 'places the needs of children and young people first, ensures they are listened to and understand decisions which affect them' (Scottish Government 2009). It builds from universal health and education services and drives the developments that will improve outcomes for children and young people. The aim is to do this by changing the way adults think and act to help all children and young people. 'It requires a positive shift in culture, systems and practice across services for children, young people and adults' (Scottish Executive 2005a, p.3).

So if we are looking at a public health approach, we might see a range of interventions that happen along a continuum and this can be a useful way to conceptualize approaches. It is entirely congruent with other models of child protection (e.g. Hardiker, Exton and Barker 1991, where a continuum of need requires a continuum of services), but offers a coherent perspective that allows multiple strategies at many different levels to be captured usefully. It has also been tested extensively across a range of needs, disease and deficit. And it is inherently interdisciplinary.

At the time of writing the Government is consulting on its public health strategy for England (HM Government 2011), urging transparency in outcomes. While focused primarily at a health audience (reflected in much of the language), it does include child protection measures within the proposals:

> Child protection services will also be able to work more closely with public health within local government. Safeguarding duties will of course continue to apply to health services commissioned under the new arrangements for local government. (Para 3.23)

The White Paper suggests that a public health outcomes framework should be organized within five domains, all of which may be useful in thinking about interventions for neglect:

1. *Health protection and resilience*: actively bolstering protective factors and increasing resilience should be core activities in neglect.

2. *Address the wider determinants of ill health*: the wider social context, the stresses and environments, are key in neglect and we need to pay attention to them.

3. *Health improvement, adoption of health lifestyles*: while this domain focuses on a traditional health promotion model and does put the onus on the individual, it still has an important message for neglect. If parents were to stop taking drugs, for example, it would be an enormous help for many children.

4. *Prevention of ill health*: where factors are preventable, we need to be working actively at making sure they are prevented. For example, stopping the cumulative harm that occurs when children experience multiple oscillations between care at home or away from home (Bromfield *et al.* 2010).

5. *Healthy life expectancy and preventable mortality*: neglect is preventable, children do not have to die from neglect, children do not have to suffer the long-term consequences of neglect. Sometimes we might need to remind ourselves of that.

We should not forget that we do know quite a lot about what prevents child maltreatment, albeit we have not always uncoupled abuse from neglect. A systematic review of reviews by Mikton and Butchart (2009) demonstrates that of five main types of prevention intervention that could be used in neglect (home visiting, parent education, multi-component interventions, media-based interventions, and support and mutual aid groups), three show promise in actually reducing child neglect (home visiting, parent education and multi-component interventions) and two of them (home visiting and parent education) appear effective in reducing risk factors for maltreatment. Methodological difficulties aside, the limitations do not undermine the main conclusions (Mikton and Butchart 2009).

Figure 6.4 explores some potential intervention points for neglect specifically. While this is presented as a bell curve, this is for illustrative purposes only. A range of interventions that take place along a continuum can be a useful way to conceptualize approaches. Our current position is a curve heavily weighted towards the downstream end. In the long term this should be reversed, with the main balance of preventive interventions at the upstream end.

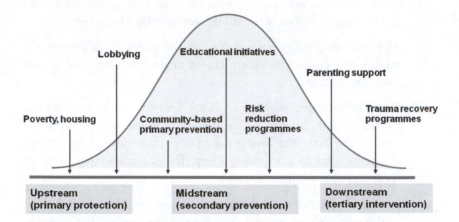

Figure 6.4: Possible points of intervention (a public health approach to neglect)

Applied to neglect this model begins to suggest a range of interventions at each level which are described below (see also Box 6.3).

Primary protection level
Universal interventions aimed at whole populations and promoting changes in societal and cultural norms and attitudes, including:

- encouraging breastfeeding for nutrition and promoting secure attachments
- establishing online safety programmes
- providing child and family health nurses for all families with a new baby, to check health and development, promote safe practices and good parenting, make referrals if required for extra needs.

Secondary prevention level
Interventions targeted at vulnerable or at-risk individuals or groups, including:

- providing support groups for children of drug-using parents
- services for adults with mental health or addiction problems noticing when there are children in the family
- offering services for teenage mothers.

Tertiary intervention level

Also known as tertiary prevention, child protection and therapeutic services to children who have already been neglected, including:

- working together with children and mothers following domestic abuse

- promoting swift decisions about safe reunification or permanent care for neglected children

- providing accessible treatment services.

Box 6.3: Activity – Thinking about preventing neglect

Consider the following three studies that were included in the systematic review. For each of them think about whether they are upstream, downstream or somewhere in the middle. Is there any way the research or the results could be scaled up to be more upstream? If they were, what would be the effects – on child neglect, and on society as a whole? What policies and actions would need to be in place for this to happen?

Parents of new-born babies were asked to complete a measure of parenting concerns. Some of them indicated they were worried that either they themselves or the baby's father might neglect them (Combs-Orme *et al.* 2004).

A longitudinal study of families on a programme to support at-risk families found that families were twice as likely to have neglect reported where there was also domestic abuse in the household (McGuigan and Pratt 2001).

One of the LONGSCAN studies (Dubowitz *et al.* 2004) showed that psychological neglect was associated with teacher report of problems in peer relationships at age six.

Conclusion

The premise of our systematic review was noticing and responding to the neglected child. As we discussed in Chapter 1, while often used interchangeably, there is a world of difference between the two. On a public health spectrum, both of these actions could be undertaken at a range of points, although responding to a child who is already neglected is clearly a more downstream activity than noticing a child who is on the verge of experiencing neglect and supporting the family to make effective changes. We believe it is possible to shift the balance in child neglect, albeit it will take huge commitment and will probably take some time. A public health approach probably offers the most coherent and systematic chance of success.

> The world is a dangerous place to live. Not because of the people who are evil, but because of the people who don't do anything about it. (Albert Einstein)

KEY MESSAGES

1. It is possible to prevent child neglect.
2. Public health approaches offer a useful framework for working with neglect.
3. We know more now than we ever have about the causes and consequences and costs of neglect.
4. We are beginning to acquire an evidence base about appropriate interventions – and these should be articulated across a public health spectrum.
5. Early intervention means early in life, early recognition, and early response.
6. Public health approaches are not the responsibility of health services.
7. Success in primary prevention appears to be a 'non-event' but in fact is a huge event.
8. Primary prevention entails adopting universal population-wide approaches.
9. Secondary prevention involves targeting intervention on sub-groups of the population where there are factors known to elevate risk of neglect.
10. Tertiary prevention aims to prevent the likelihood of poor outcomes as a result of a child having experienced neglect.

Appendix 1

Systematic Review Methodology

The method was based on systematic review guidelines issued by the University of York NHS Centre for Reviews and Dissemination (Centre for Reviews and Dissemination 2007).

Search aims

We aimed to locate national and international primary research studies, theoretical papers and reviews published in English from 1995–2005 that described or analysed:

- the views of children, parents and the general public about the features of professional systems that facilitate access to appropriate help
- the characteristics of parents (including male figures and substitute carers), and of their behaviour, directly or indirectly associated with child neglect
- 'proxy' indications of the potential for neglect such as parental substance misuse, domestic abuse and parental mental health problems
- the signs in children, parents and in the relationship between the two that indicate that intervention is required
- the ways in which different agencies and professions operationalize neglect and sub-types of neglect
- recognition and detection of neglect by any lay or professional group
- different arrangements for interagency communication and collaboration and their effectiveness for swift response to children's unmet needs including thresholds for action
- self-referral by children or parents

- the ways in which children and parents directly and indirectly signal their need for help

- the characteristics of services that are accessible to families where there is risk of child neglect

- the needs of Black and ethnic minority children and their families

- the needs of disabled children.

Search strategy

This was an interdisciplinary piece of research focusing on an area where a large variety of professionals such as police, paediatricians, social workers, nurses and speech therapists could be involved. Therefore bibliographic databases which cover published literature concerning these and other fields were interrogated. This included CINAHL, EmBase, MEDLINE, PsycINFO and ERIC among others.

Studies eligible for inclusion included those that:

- focused directly on children aged from pre-birth to 19 only, on the parents only, or on both parents and children

- covered the spectrum of those considered 'at risk' of neglect through to those subject to statutory provisions as a result of neglect

- involved adults who were neglected as children

- examined the response of professionals to neglected children and their families

- identified specific criteria for identification and selection into neglect prevention programmes

- identified specific criteria for neglect treatment programmes.

Studies and papers not eligible for inclusion in the final dataset were those:

- that aimed specifically at intervention after neglect and treatment of children or parents

- where different forms of abuse and neglect were conflated (except where the findings were particularly relevant to the topic).

Screening and filtering

The rigorous filtering process that culled an initial 20,480 potentially relevant articles to a final data set of 63 is summarized in Figure A.1:

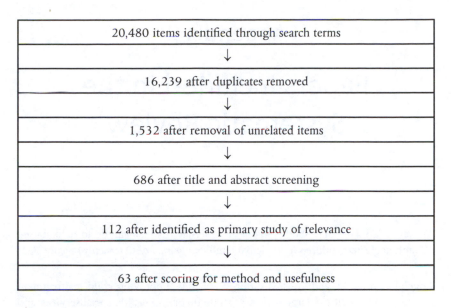

Figure A.1: Showing the filtering process

Final inclusion and data extraction

Each study was read in full by one member of the team using a data extraction form to collate standardized information. Our quality ratings for the studies were based on widely available critical appraisal tools, whereby we gave a methodological score to all fully appraised papers ($n = 112$) based on a standardized assessment. A three-point scale was used: 1 – we were confident that the research was rigorously designed and undertaken, and potential bias had been addressed; we were satisfied with the overall design and methods, and attempts to address bias had been taken, or at the very least, acknowledged. Studies that were assigned a 3 rating did not satisfy our basic criteria of rigour, or were flawed in some other way, or bias had not been addressed.

We also used a three-point rating scale to establish how useful a paper was in answering our research question. Papers were scored: 1 – extremely useful and directly relevant to the research question, providing insight into practitioner recognition of and response to child neglect; 2 – some useful information about neglect, but not directly relevant; 3 – very little (if anything) of relevance to the research question.

Appendix 2

Papers Included in the Systematic Review

Andrews, A.B. (1996) 'Public opinions about what a citizen can do to help abused and neglected children in addictive families.' *Journal of Community Practice, 3,* 1, 19–33.

Angeles Cerezo, M. and Pons-Salvador, G. (2004) 'Improving child maltreatment detection systems: A large-scale case study involving health, social services, and school professionals.' *Child Abuse and Neglect, 28,* 1153–1170.

Appleton, J.V. (1996) 'Working with vulnerable families: A health visiting perspective.' *Journal of Advanced Nursing, 23,* 5, 912–918.

Appleton, J.V. and Cowley, S. (2004) 'The guideline contradiction: Health visitors' use of formal guidelines for identifying and assessing families in need.' *International Journal of Nursing Studies, 41,* 7, 785–797.

Ashton, V. (2004) 'The effect of personal characteristics on reporting child maltreatment.' *Child Abuse and Neglect: The International Journal, 28,* 9, 985–997.

Atta, H.Y. and Youssef, R.M. (1998) 'Child abuse and neglect: Mothers' behaviour and perceptions.' *Eastern Mediterranean Health Journal, 4,* 3, 502–512.

Ayre, P. (1998) 'Assessment of significant harm: Improving professional practice.' *British Journal of Nursing, 7,* 1, 31–36.

Barlow J., Davis H., McIntosh E., Jarrett P., Mockford C. and Stewart-Brown S. (2007) 'Role of home visiting in improving parenting and health in families at risk of abuse and neglect: Results of a multicentre randomised controlled trial and economic evaluation.' *Archives of Disease in Childhood, 92,* 3, 229–233.

Brown J., Cohen P., Johnson, J.G. and Salzinger, S. (1998) 'A longitudinal analysis of risk factors for child maltreatment: Findings of a 17-year prospective study of officially recorded and self-reported child abuse and neglect.' *Child Abuse and Neglect, 22,* 11, 1065–1078.

Bryant, A.A. (2000) 'Enhancing parent-child interaction with a prenatal couple intervention.' *The American Journal of Maternal/Child Nursing, 25,* 3, 139–145.

Carpenter, M., Kennedy, M., Armstrong, A.L. and Moore, E. (1997) 'Indicators of abuse or neglect in preschool children's drawings.' *Journal of Psychosocial Nursing and Mental Health Services, 35*, 4, 10–17.

Carter, V. and Myers, M.R. (2007) 'Exploring the risks of substantiated physical neglect related to poverty and parental characteristics: A national sample.' *Children and Youth Services Review, 29*, 110–121.

Cash, S.J. and Wilke, D.J. (2003) 'An ecological model of maternal substance abuse and child neglect: Issues, analyses, and recommendations.' *American Journal of Orthopsychiatry, 73*, 4, 392–404.

Chester, D.L., Jose, R.M., Aldlyami, E., King, H. and Moiemen, N.S. (2006) 'Non-accidental burns in children: Are we neglecting neglect?' *Burns, 32*, 2, 222–228.

Christensen, E. (1999) 'The prevalence and nature of abuse and neglect in children under four: A national survey.' *Child Abuse Review, 8*, 2, 109–119.

Combs-Orme, T., Cain, D.S. and Wilson, E.E. (2004) 'Do maternal concerns at delivery predict parenting stress during infancy?' *Child Abuse and Neglect, 28*, 377–392.

Connell-Carrick, K. and Scannapieco, M. (2006) 'Ecological correlates of neglect in infants and toddlers.' *Journal of Interpersonal Violence, 21*, 3, 299–316.

Coohey, C. and Zhang Y. (2006) 'The role of men in chronic supervisory neglect.' *Child Maltreatment, 11*, 1, 27–33.

Daniel, B. (2000) 'Judgements about parenting: What do social workers think they are doing?' *Child Abuse Review*, Mar-Apr, 91–107.

Depaul, J. and Arruabarrena, M.I. (1995) 'Behavior problems in school-aged physically abused and neglected children in Spain.' *Child Abuse and Neglect, 19*, 4, 409–418.

Dubowitz, H., Black, M.M., Kerr, M.A., Starr, R.H., Jr. and Harrington, D. (2000) 'Fathers and child neglect.' *Archives of Pediatrics and Adolescent Medicine, 154*, 2, 135–141.

Dubowitz, H., Klockner, A., Starr, R.H., Jr. and Black, M.M. (1998) 'Community and professional definitions of child neglect.' *Child Maltreatment, 3*, 3, 235–243.

Dubowitz, H., Papas, M.A., Black, M.M. and Starr, R.H. (2002) 'Child neglect: Outcomes in high-risk urban preschoolers.' *Pediatrics, 109*, 6, 1100–1107.

Dubowitz, H., Pitts, S.C. and Black, M.M. (2004) 'Measurement of three major subtypes of child neglect.' *Child Maltreatment, 9*, 4, 344–356.

Dubowitz, H., Pitts, S.C., Litrownik, A.J., Cox, C.E., Runyan, D.K. and Black, M. (2005) 'Defining child neglect based on child protective services data.' *Child Abuse and Neglect, 29*, 5, 493–512.

English, D.J., Thompson, R., Graham, J.C. and Briggs, E.C. (2005) 'Toward a definition of neglect in young children.' *Child Maltreatment, 10*, 2, 190–206.

Friedlaender, E.Y., Rubin, D.M., Alpern, E.R., Mandell, D.S., Christian, C.W. and Alessandrini, E.A. (2005) 'Patterns of health care use that may identify young children who are at risk for maltreatment.' *Pediatrics, 116,* 6, 1303–1308.

Gaudin, J.M., Polansky, N.A., Kilpatrick, A.C. and Shilton, P. (1996) 'Family functioning in neglectful families.' *Child Abuse and Neglect, 20,* 4, 363–377.

Gillham, B., Tanner, G., Cheyne, B., Freeman, I., Rooney, M. and Lambie, A. (1998) 'Unemployment rates, single parent density, and indices of child poverty: Their relationship to different categories of child abuse and neglect.' *Child Abuse and Neglect, 22,* 2, 79–90.

Hansen, D.J., Bumby, K.M., Lundquist, L.M., Chandler, R.M., Le, P.T. and Futa, K.T. (1997) 'The influence of case and professional variables on the identification and reporting of child maltreatment: A study of licensed psychologists and certified masters social workers.' *Journal of Family Violence, 12,* 3, 313–332.

Harrington, D., Black, M.M., Starr, R.H., Jr. and Dubowitz, H. (1998) 'Child neglect: Relation to child temperament and family context.' *American Journal of Orthopsychiatry, 68,* 1, 108–116.

Harrington, D., Dubowitz, H., Black, M.M. and Binder, A. (1995) 'Maternal substance use and neglectful parenting: Relations with children's development.' *Journal of Clinical Child Psychology, 24,* 3, 258–263.

Hines, D.A., Kantor, G.K. and Holt, M.K. (2006) 'Similarities in siblings' experiences of neglectful parenting behaviors.' *Child Abuse and Neglect, 30,* 6, 619–637.

Hultman, C.S., Priolo, D., Cairns, B.A., Grant, E.J., Peterson, H.D. and Meyer, A.A. (1998) 'Psychosocial forum. Return to jeopardy: The fate of pediatric burn patients who are victims of abuse and neglect... including commentary by Doctor M.' *Journal of Burn Care and Rehabilitation, 19,* 4, 367–376.

Jaudes, P., Ekwo, E. and VanVoorhis, J. (1995) 'Association of drug abuse and child abuse.' *Child Abuse and Neglect, 19,* 1065–1075.

Kantor, G.K., Holt, M.K., Mebert, C.J., Straus, M.A., Drach, K.M., Ricci, L.R., *et al.* (2004) 'Development and preliminary psychometric properties of the Multidimensional Neglectful Behavior Scale-Child Report.' *Child Maltreatment, 9,* 4, 409–428.

Lagerberg, D. (2004) 'A descriptive survey of Swedish child health nurses' awareness of abuse and neglect. II. Characteristics of the children.' *Acta Paediatrica, 93,* 5, 692–701.

Lewin, D. and Herron, H. (2007) 'Signs, symptoms and risk factors: Health visitors' perspectives of child neglect.' *Child Abuse Review, 16,* 93–107.

Ling, M.S. and Luker, K.A. (2000) 'Protecting children: Intuition and awareness in the work of health visitors.' *Journal of Advanced Nursing, 32,* 3, 572–579.

MacMillan, H.L., Thomas, B.H., Jamieson, E., Walsh, C.A., Boyle, M.H., Shannon, H.S., *et al.* (2005) 'Effectiveness of home visitation by public-health nurses in prevention of the recurrence of child physical abuse and neglect: A randomised controlled trial.' *Lancet, 365*, 9473, 1786–1793.

Maiter, S., Alaggia, R. and Trocme, N. (2004) 'Perceptions of child maltreatment by parents from the Indian subcontinent: challenging myths about culturally based abusive parenting practices.' *Child Maltreatment, 9*, 3, 309–324.

May-Chahal, C. and Cawson, P. (2005) 'Measuring child maltreatment in the United Kingdom: A study of the prevalence of child abuse and neglect.' *Child Abuse and Neglect, 29*, 9, 969–984.

McGuigan, W.M. and Pratt, C.C. (2001) 'The predictive impact of domestic violence on three types of child maltreatment.' *Child Abuse and Neglect, 25*, 7, 869–883.

McKeganey, N., Barnard, M. and McIntosh, J. (2002) 'Paying the price for their parents' addiction: Meeting the needs of the children of drug-using parents.' *Drugs: Education, Prevention and Policy, 9*, 3, 233–246.

Mitchell, L.M., Turbiville, V. and Turnbull, H.R., III. (1999) 'Reporting abuse and neglect of children with disabilities: Early childhood service providers' views.' *Infants and Young Children, 11*, 3, 19–26.

Nair, P., Black, M.M., Schuler, M., Keane, V., Snow, L., Rigney, B.A., *et al.* (1997) 'Risk factors for disruption in primary caregiving among infants of substance abusing women.' *Child Abuse and Neglect, 21*, 11, 1039–1051.

Nair, P., Schuler, M.E., Blacka, M.M., Kettinger, L. and Harrington, D. (2003) 'Cumulative environmental risk in substance abusing women: Early intervention, parenting stress, child abuse potential and child development.' *Child Abuse and Neglect, 27*, 9, 997–1017.

Narayan, A.P., Socolar, R.R.S. and St Claire, K. (2006) 'Pediatric residency training in child abuse and neglect in the United States.' *Pediatrics, 117*, 6, 2215–2221.

Ondersma, S.J. (2002) 'Predictors of neglect within low-SES families: The importance of substance abuse.' *American Journal of Orthopsychiatry, 72*, 3, 383–391.

Paavilainen, E., Astedt-Kurki, P. and Paunonen, M. (2000) 'School nurses' operational modes and ways of collaborating in caring for child abusing families in Finland.' *Journal of Clinical Nursing, 9*, 5, 742–750.

Paavilainen, E., Merikanto, J., Astedt-Kurki, P., Laippala, P., Tammentie, T. and Paunonen-Ilmonen, M. (2002) 'Identification of child maltreatment while caring for them in a university hospital.' *International Journal of Nursing Studies, 39*, 3, 287–294.

Paavilainen, E. and Tarkka, M. (2003) 'Definition and identification of child abuse by Finnish public health nurses.' *Public Health Nursing, 20*, 1, 49–55.

Rose, S.J. (1999) 'Reaching consensus on child neglect: African American mothers and child welfare workers.' *Children and Youth Services Review, 21*, 6, 463–479.

Rose, S.J. and Meezan, W. (1996) 'Variations in perceptions of child neglect.' *Child Welfare Journal, 75,* 2, 139–160.

Rose, S.J. and Selwyn, J. (2000) 'Child neglect: An English perspective.' *International Social Work, 43,* 2, 179–192.

Scannapieco, M. and Connell-Carrick, K. (2003) 'Families in poverty: Those who maltreat their infants and toddlers and those who do not.' *Journal of Family Social Work, 7,* 3, 49–70.

Scannapieco, M. and Connell-Carrick, K. (2005) 'Focus on the First Years: Correlates of Substantiation of Child Maltreatment for Families with Children 0 to 4.' *Children and Youth Services Review 27,* 1307–1323.

Sheehan, R. (2004) 'Partnership in mental health and child welfare: Social work responses to children living with parental mental illness.' *Social Work in Health Care, 39,* 3/4, 309–324.

Thyen, U., Leventhal, J.M., Yazdgerdi, S.R. and Perrin, J.M. (1997) 'Concerns about Child Maltreatment in Hospitalized Children.' *Child Abuse and Neglect: The International Journal, 21,* 2, 187–198.

Vincent, S. and Daniel, B. (2004) 'An analysis of children and young people's calls to ChildLine about abuse and neglect: A study for the Scottish child protection review.' *Child Abuse Review, 13,* 2, 158–171.

Wiklund, S. (2006) 'Signs of child maltreatment: The extent and nature of referrals to Swedish child welfare agencies.' *European Journal of Social Work, 9,* 1, 39–58.

Wilding, J. and Thoburn, J. (1997) 'Family support plans for neglected and emotionally maltreated children.' *Child Abuse Review, 6,* 5, 343–356.

Wright, C. and Birks, E. (2000) 'Risk factors for failure to thrive: A population-based survey.' *Child: Care, Health and Development,* Jan, 5–16.

References

Action for Children (2010) *Seen and Now Heard: Taking Action on Child Neglect.* London: Action for Children.

Aldgate, J. and Rose, W. (2008) *Assessing and Managing Risk in Getting it Right for Every Child.* Edinburgh: Scottish Government.

Aldgate, J. and Statham, J. (2001) *The Children Act Now: Messages from Research.* London: The Stationery Office.

Aldridge, J. and Becker, S. (2003) *Children Who Care for Parents with Mental Illness: The Perspectives of Young Carers, Parents and Professionals.* London: Policy Press.

American Academy of Pediatric Dentistry (2003) 'Definition of dental neglect.' *Pediatr Dent., 25 (suppl),* 13.

Anda, R. and Felitti, V. (2010) 'The Adverse Childhood Experiences (ACE) Study [online].' Available at www.acestudy.org, accessed on 2 June 2010.

Andrews, A.B. (1996) 'Public opinions about what a citizen can do to help abused and neglected children in addictive families.' *Journal of Community Practice, 3,* 1, 19–33.

Angeles Cerezo, M. and Pons-Salvador, G. (2004) 'Improving child maltreatment detection systems: A large-scale case study involving health, social services, and school professionals.' *Child Abuse and Neglect, 28,* 1153–1170.

Anning, A., Stuart, J., Nicholls, M., Goldthorpe, J. and Morley, A. (2007) *Understanding Variations in Effectiveness Amongst Sure Start Local Programmes: Final Report.* London: DfES.

Appleton, J.V. (1996) 'Working with vulnerable families: A health visiting perspective.' *Journal of Advanced Nursing, 23,* 5, 912–918.

Appleton, J.V. and Cowley, S. (2004) 'The guideline contradiction: Health visitors' use of formal guidelines for identifying and assessing families in need.' *International Journal of Nursing Studies, 41,* 7, 785–797.

Arcia, E. and Fernandez, M.C. (1998) 'Cuban mothers' schemas of ADHD: Development, characteristics and help seeking behaviour. ' *Journal of Child and Family Studies, 7,* 333–352.

Ashton, V. (2004) 'The effect of personal characteristics on reporting child maltreatment.' *Child Abuse and Neglect: The International Journal, 28,* 9, 985–997.

Atta, H.Y. and Youssef, R.M. (1998) 'Child abuse and neglect: Mothers' behaviour and perceptions.' *Eastern Mediterranean Health Journal, 4,* 3, 502–512.

Austin, M. and Priest, S. (2004) 'New developments in perinatal mental health.' *Acta Psychiatrica Scandinavica, 110*, 321–322.

Baginsky, M. (2000) *Child Protection and Education.* London: NSPCC.

Baginsky, M. (2003) 'Newly Qualified Teachers and Child Protection: A Survey of Their Views.' *Child Abuse Review, 12*, 119–127.

Baginsky, M. (ed.) (2008) *Safeguarding Children and Schools.* London: Jessica Kingsley Publishers.

Baker-Henningham, H., Powell, C., Walker, S. and Grantham-McGregor, S. (2005) 'The effect of early stimulation on maternal depression: A cluster randomised controlled trial.' *Archives of Disease in Childhood, 90*, 1230–1234.

Barlow, J. (2008) *Setting the Scene. A Public Health Approach to Child Protection* (*conference report*). London: NSPCC. Available at www.nspcc.org.uk/Inform/ newsandevents/ConferenceReports/SettingTheScene_wdf60476.pdf, accessed 14 March 2011.

Barlow, J. and Schrader-MacMillan, A. (2009) *Safeguarding Children from Emotional Abuse – What Works?* (*Research Brief*). London: Department for Education.

Barlow, J. with Scott, J. (2010) *Safeguarding in the 21st Century: Where to Now?* Totness: Research in Practice.

Barnard, M. and Barlow, J. (2003) 'Discovering parental drug dependence: Silence and disclosure.' *Children and Society, 17*, 45–56.

Belgrave, M., Jakob-Hoff, M., Milne, S., Selby, R., Asiasiger, L., Mataira, P., *et al.* (2002) *Social Workers in Schools, Expansion Evaluation, Final Report.* Wellington, NZ: Ministry of Social Development.

Benard, B. (2004) *Resiliency: What Have We Learned?* San Francisco, CA: WestEd.

Berry, M., Charlston, R. and Dawson, K. (2003) 'Promising practices in understanding and treating child neglect.' *Child and Family Social Work, 8*, 1, 13–24.

Black, M.M., Dubowitz, H., Krishnakumar, A. and Starr, R.H. (2007) 'Early intervention and recovery among children with failure to thrive: Follow-up at age 8.' *Pediatrics, 120*, 1, 59–69.

Brandon, M., Belderson, P., Warren, C., Howe, D., Garnder, R., Dodsworth, J., *et al.* (2008) *Analysing Child Deaths and Serious Injury Through Abuse and Neglect: What Can We Learn? A Biennial Analysis of Serious Case Reviews 2003–2005.* London: DCSF.

Broadhurst, K. (2003) 'Engaging parents and carers with family support services: What can be learned from research on help-seeking?' *Child and Family Social Work, 8*, 341–350.

Bromfield, L., Lamont, A., Parker, R. and Horsfall, B. (2010) 'Issues for the safety and wellbeing of children in families with multiple and complex problems. The co-occurrence of domestic violence, parental substance misuse, and mental health problems.' *NPC Issues, 33*, 1–23.

Bromfield, L. and Miller, R. (2007) *Specialist Practice Guide: Cumulative Harm.* Melbourne, Australia: State Government Victoria Department of Human Services.

Brown, J., Cohen, P., Johnson, J.G. and Salzinger, S. (1998) 'A longitudinal analysis of risk factors for child maltreatment: Findings of a 17-year prospective study of officially recorded and self-reported child abuse and neglect.' *Child Abuse and Neglect, 22*, 11, 1065–1078.

Browne, K., Hamilton-Giachritis, C. and Vettor, S. (2007) *Preventing Child Maltreatment in Europe: A Public Health Approach.* Copenhagen, Denmark: WHO.

Brunk, M., Henggeler, S.W. and Whelan, J.P. (1987) 'Comparison of Multisystemic Therapy and Parent Training in the brief treatment of child abuse and neglect.' *Journal of Clinical and Consulting Psychology, 55*, 171–178.

Bryant, J. and Milsom, A. (2005) 'Child abuse reporting by school counselors.' *Professional School Counseling, 9*, 1, 63–71.

Buckley, H. (2005) 'Neglect: No Monopoly on Expertise.' In J. Taylor and B. Daniels (eds) *Child Neglect: Practice Issues for Health and Social Care.* London: Jessica Kingsley Publishers..

Burke, J., Chandy, J., Dannerbeck, A. and Watt, J.W. (1998) 'The parental cluster model of child neglect: An integrative conceptual model.' *Child Welfare, 77*, 4, 389–405.

Burke, K. and Gruenert, S. (2005) *Parenting Support Toolkit for Alcohol and Other Drug Workers.* Melbourne, Australia: Victorian Government Department of Human Services.

Butchart, A., Harvey, A.P. and Fumiss, T. (2006) *Preventing Child Maltreatment: A Guide to Taking Action and Generating Evidence.* Geneva, Switzerland: WHO and ISPCAN.

C4EO (2009) *Grasping the Nettle: Early Intervention for Children, Families and Communities.* London: Centre for Excellence and Outcomes in Children and Young People's Services (C4EO).

Cabinet Office (2007a) *Reaching Out: An Action Plan on Social Exclusion.* London: Cabinet Office.

Cabinet Office (2007b) *Reaching Out: Think Family Analysis and Themes from the Families At Risk Review.* London: Cabinet Office.

Carpenter, J., Hackett, S., Patsios, D. and Szilassy, E. (2010) *Outcomes of Interagency Training to Safeguard Children: Final Report to the Department for Children, Schools and Families and the Department of Health.* London: DfE.

Carpenter, M., Kennedy, M., Armstrong, A.L. and Moore, E. (1997) 'Indicators of abuse or neglect in preschool children's drawings.' *Journal of Psychosocial Nursing and Mental Health Services, 35*, 4, 10–17.

Carter, V. and Myers, M.R. (2007) 'Exploring the risks of substantiated physical neglect related to poverty and parental characteristics: A national sample.' *Children and Youth Services Review, 29,* 110–121.

Cash, S.J. and Wilke, D.J. (2003) 'An ecological model of maternal substance abuse and child neglect: Issues, analyses, and recommendations.' *American Journal of Orthopsychiatry, 73,* 4, 392–404.

Centre for Reviews and Dissemination (2007) *Review Methods and Resources.* York: University of York.

Chester, D.L., Jose, R.M., Aldlyami, E., King, H. and Moiemen, N.S. (2006) 'Non-accidental burns in children: Are we neglecting neglect?' *Burns, 32,* 2, 222–228.

Children, Youth and Families Act (2005) Victoria, Australia: State Government of Victoria.

Cleaver, H. and Freeman, P. (1995) *Parent Perspectives in Cases of Suspected Child Abuse.* London: HMSO.

Cleaver, H., Nicholson, D., Tarr, S. and Cleaver, D. (2006) *The Response of Child Protection Practices and Procedures to Children Exposed to Domestic Violence or Parental Substance Misuse: Executive Summary.* London: DfES.

Cleaver, H., Unell, I. and Aldgate, J. (1999) *Children's Needs – Parenting Capacity: The Impact of Parental Mental Illness, Problem Alcohol and Drugs Use, and Domestic Violence on the Development of Children.* London: The Stationery Office.

Cleaver, H., Walker, S. and Meadows, P. (2004) *Assessing Children's Needs and Circumstances: The Impact of the Assessment Framework.* London: Jessica Kingsley Publishers.

Combs-Orme, T., Cain, D.S. and Wilson, E.E. (2004) 'Do maternal concerns at delivery predict parenting stress during infancy?' *Child Abuse and Neglect, 28,* 377–392.

Connell-Carrick, K. and Scannapieco, M. (2006) 'Ecological correlates of neglect in infants and toddlers.' *Journal of Interpersonal Violence, 21,* 3, 299–316.

Coohey, C. (1998) 'Home alone and other inadequately supervised children.' *Child Welfare, 77,* 3, 291–310.

Coohey, C. and Zhang, Y. (2006) 'The role of men in chronic supervisory neglect.' *Child Maltreatment, 11,* 1, 27–33.

Cooper, A., Hetherington, R. and Katz, I. (2003) *The Risk Factor: Making the Child Protection System Work for Children.* London: DEMOS.

Cowan, P. and Cowan, C. (2008) 'Diverging family policies to promote children's well-being in the UK and US: Some relevant data from family research and intervention studies.' *Journal of Children's Services, 3,* 4, 4–16.

CRAE (2003) *Let Them Have Their Childhood Again.* London: Children's Rights Alliance for England.

Crittenden, P.M. (1996) 'Research on Maltreating Families: Implications for Intervention.' In J. Briere, L. Berliner, J.A. Bulkley, C. Jenny and T. Reid (eds) *The APSAC Handbook on Child Maltreatment.* Newbury Park, London; New Delhi: Sage.

Crittenden, P.M. (1999) 'Child Neglect: Causes and Contribution.' In H. Dubowitz (ed.) *Neglected Children: Research, Practice and Policy.* London: Sage.

Daniel, B. (1999a) 'A picture of powerlessness: An exploration of child neglect and ways in which social workers and parents can be empowered towards efficacy.' *International Journal of Child and Family Welfare, 4,* 3, 209–220.

Daniel, B. (1999b) 'Beliefs in child care: Social work consensus and lack of consensus on issues of parenting and decision-making.' *Children and Society, 13,* 171–191.

Daniel, B. (2005) 'Introduction to Issues for Health and Social Care in Neglect.' In J. Taylor and B. Daniel (eds) *Neglect: Practice Issues for Health and Social Care.* London: Jessica Kingsley Publishers.

Daniel, B. and Taylor, J. (2005) 'Do they Care? The Role of Fathers in Cases of Child Neglect.' In J. Taylor and B. Daniel (eds) *Child Neglect: Practice Issues for Health and Social Care.* London: Jessica Kingsley Publishers.

Daniel, B., Vincent, S., Farrall, E. and Arney, F., (2009) 'How is the Concept of Resilience Operationalised in Practice with Vulnerable Children?' *International Journal of Child and Family Welfare, 12,* 1, 2–21.

Daniel, B. and Wassell, S. (2002) *The Early Years: Assessing and Promoting Resilience in Vulnerable Children I.* London: Jessica Kingsley Publishers.

Daro, D. (1988) *Confronting Child Abuse.* New York, NY: New York Free Press.

Daro, D. and Dodge, K. (2009) 'Creating community responsibility for child protection: Possibilities and challenges.' *The Future of Children, 19,* 2, 67–93.

DCSF (2007a) *The Children's Plan: Building Brighter Futures.* London: Department for Children, Schools and Families.

DCSF (2007b) *Staying Safe: Action Plan.* London: Department for Children, Schools and Families.

DePanfilis, D. (2006) *Child Neglect: A Guide for Prevention, Assessment and Intervention.* New York, NY: Children's Bureau, Office on Child Abuse and Neglect.

Department for Education (2010) *DfE: Children In Need in England, including their characteristics and further information on children who were the subject of a child protection plan (2009–10 Children in Need census, Final).* London: Department for Education; Department for Business, Innovation and Skills.

Department of Health (1999) *Framework for the Assessment of Children in Need and Their Families (Consultation Draft).* London: Department of Health.

Department of Health (2000) *Framework for the Assessment of Children in Need and their Families.* London: The Stationery Office.

Department of Health (2002) *Safeguarding Children: A Joint Chief Inspectors' Report on Arrangements to Safeguard Children.* London: Department of Health.

Department of Health (2004) *National Service Framework for Children, Young People and Maternity Services.* London: Department of Health.

Department of Health (2006) *Child Protection and the Dental Team.* Available at www. cpdt.org.uk/index.htm, accessed on 8 January 2011.

Department of Health, Home Office, and Department for Education and Employment. (1999) *Working Together to Safeguard Children.* London: The Stationery Office.

Department of Health, Home Office, and DFES (2003) *Keeping Children Safe: The Government's Response to the Victoria Climbié Report and Joint Chief Inspectors' Report Safeguarding Children.* London: The Stationery Office.

Depaul, J. and Arruabarrena, M.I. (1995) 'Behavior problems in school-aged physically abused and neglected children in Spain.' *Child Abuse and Neglect, 19,* 4, 409–418.

DFES (2004) *Every Child Matters: Change for Children.* London: The Stationery Office.

Dingwall, R., Eekelaar, J. and Murray, T. (1995) *The Protection of Children: State Intervention and Family Life* (2nd edition). Oxford: Blackwell.

Doyle, C. (2007) 'Child protection and child outcomes: Measuring the effects of foster care.' *American Economic Review, 97,* 5, 1583–1610.

Dubowitz, H., Black, M.M., Kerr, M.A., Starr, R.H., Jr. and Harrington, D. (2000) 'Fathers and child neglect.' *Archives of Pediatrics and Adolescent Medicine, 154,* 2, 135–141.

Dubowitz, H., Klockner, A., Starr, R.H., Jr. and Black, M.M. (1998) 'Community and professional definitions of child neglect.' *Child Maltreatment, 3,* 3, 235–243.

Dubowitz, H., Papas, M.A., Black, M.M. and Starr, R.H. (2002) 'Child neglect: Outcomes in high-risk urban preschoolers.' *Pediatrics, 109,* 6, 1100–1107.

Dubowitz, H., Pitts, S.C. and Black, M.M. (2004) 'Measurement of three major subtypes of child neglect.' *Child Maltreatment, 9,* 4, 344–356.

Duncan, S. and Reder, P. (2000) 'Children's Experience of Major Psychiatric Disorder in their Parent: An Overview.' In P. Reder, McClure, M. and A. Jolley (eds) *Family Matters: Interfaces between Child and Adult Mental Health.* London: Routledge.

Edwards, J. (1995) '"Parenting skills": Views of community health and social service providers about the needs of their "clients".' *Journal of Social Policy, 24,* 2, 237–259.

Egeland, B. (1991) 'A longitudinal study of high risk families: Issues and findings.' In R.H. Starr and D.A. Wolfe (eds) *The Effects of Child Abuse and Neglect. Issues and Research.* New York, NY: Guilford Press.

Egeland, B., Sroufe, L.A. and Erickson, M. (1983) 'The developmental consequences of different patterns of maltreatment.' *Child Abuse and Neglect, 7,* 459–469.

English, D.J., Thompson, R., Graham, J.C. and Briggs, E.C. (2005) 'Toward a definition of neglect in young children.' *Child Maltreatment, 10,* 2, 190–206.

Ewart, S. (2003) *An Investigation into the Involvement of Fathers in Family Centre Social Work in Northern Ireland.* Ulster, NI: University of Ulster, Magee.

Farmer, E. and Lutman, E. (2010) *Case Management and Outcomes for Neglected Children Returned to their Parents: A Five Year Follow-Up Study (Research Brief).* London: Department for Education.

Faugier, J. and Sargeant, M. (1997) 'Sampling hard to reach populations.' *Journal of Advanced Nursing, 26,* 790–797.

Forehand, R. and Kotchik, B. (2002) 'Behavioural Parent Training: Current Challenges and Potential Solutions.' *Journal of Child and Family Studies, 11,* 377–383.

Forrester, D. (2000) 'Parental substance misuse and child protection in a British sample. A survey of children on the child protection register in an Inner London District Office.' *Child Abuse Review, 9,* 235–246.

France, A., Munro, E.R. and Waring, A. (2010) *Effective Operation of the New Local Safeguarding Children Boards in England – Final Report.* London: Department for Education.

Friedlaender, E.Y., Rubin, D.M., Alpern, E.R., Mandell, D.S., Christian, C.W. and Alessandrini, E.A. (2005) 'Patterns of health care use that may identify young children who are at risk for maltreatment.' *Pediatrics, 116,* 6, 1303–1308.

Garbarino, G., Vorrasi, J.A. and Kostelny, K. (2002) 'Parenting and Public Policy.' In M.H. Bornstein (ed.) *Handbook of Parenting Vol. 5, Practical Issues in Parenting.* New Jersey, NJ: Laurence Erlbaum Associates.

Gardner, R. (2010) *Scoping Report: Neglect.* London: NSPCC.

Garrison, M. (2005) 'Reforming child protection: A public health perspective.' *Virginia Journal of Social Policy and the Law, 46,* 2–52.

Gaudin, J. (1993a) 'Effective interventions with neglectful families.' *Criminal Justice and Behavior, 20,* 66–89.

Gaudin, J.M. (1993b) *Child Neglect: A Guide for Intervention.* Washington DC: National Center on Child Abuse and Neglect (US Department of Health and Human Services).

Gaudin, J.M., Polansky, N.A., Kilpatrick, A.C. and Shilton, P. (1996) 'Family functioning in neglectful families.' *Child Abuse and Neglect, 20,* 4, 363–377.

Ghate, D. and Hazel, N. (2002) *Parenting in Poor Environments.* London: Jessica Kingsley Publishers.

Gilbert, R, Wilson, C.S., Browne, K., Fergusson, D.M., Webb, E. and Janson, S. (2009) 'Child maltreatment 1: Burden and consequences of child maltreatment in high-income countries.' *The Lancet, 373,* 68–81.

Gill, P. (2010) 'Baby P: What would you have done?' *Community Care, 9 November* 9, 23–25.

Gillham, B., Tanner, G., Cheyne, B., Freeman, I., Rooney, M. and Lambie, A. (1998) 'Unemployment rates, single parent density, and indices of child poverty: Their relationship to different categories of child abuse and neglect.' *Child Abuse and Neglect, 22*, 2, 79–90.

Glaser, D. (2007) 'The effects of child maltreatment on the brain.' *The Link: The Official Newsletter of the International Society for the Prevention of Child Abuse and Neglect, 16*, 2, 1–4.

Gorin, S. (2004) *Understanding What Children Say: Children's Experiences of Domestic Violence, Parental Substance Misuse and Parental Mental Health Problems. Report for the Joseph Rowntree Foundation.* London: National Children's Bureau.

Hallet, C., Murray, C. and Punch, S. (2003) 'Young People and Welfare: Negotiating Pathways.' In C. Hallet and A. Prout (eds) *Hearing the Voices of Children: Social Policy for a New Century.* London and New York, NY: Routledge Falmer.

Hansen, D.J., Bumby, K.M., Lundquist, L.M., Chandler, R.M., Le, P.T. and Futa, K.T. (1997) 'The influence of case and professional variables on the identification and reporting of child maltreatment: A study of licensed psychologists and certified masters social workers.' *Journal of Family Violence, 12*, 3, 313–332.

Hardiker, P., Exton, K. and Barker, M. (1991) 'The social policy contexts of prevention in child care.' *British Journal of Social Work, 21*, 341–359.

Harrington, D., Black, M.M., Starr, R.H., Jr. and Dubowitz, H. (1998) 'Child neglect: Relation to child temperament and family context.' *American Journal of Orthopsychiatry, 68*, 1, 108–116.

Hayden, C. and Johnson, D. (2000) *Care Proceedings in the City of Portsmouth.* University of Portsmouth: SSRIU Occasional Paper no. 51.

Helm, D. (2010) *Making Sense of Child and Family Assessment: How to Interpret Children's Needs.* London: Jessica Kingsley Publishers.

Hendry, E. (2010) *Scoping Report: Looked After Children.* London: NSPCC.

Hester, M., Pearson, C. and Harwin, N. (2007) *Making an Impact. Children and Domestic Violence. A Reader* (2nd Edition). London: Jessica Kingsley Publishers.

Hicks, L. and Stein, M. (2010) *Neglect Matters: A Multi-Agency Guide for Professionals Working Together on Behalf of Teenagers.* London: DfE.

Hines, D.A., Kantor, G.K. and Holt, M.K. (2006) 'Similarities in siblings' experiences of neglectful parenting behaviors.' *Child Abuse and Neglect, 30*, 6, 619–637.

HM Government (2010) *Working Together to Safeguard Children: A Guide to Inter-Agency Working to Safeguard and Promote the Welfare of Children.* London: HM Government.

HM Government (2011) *Healthy Lives, Healthy People.* London: The Stationary Office.

Home Office (2003) *Hidden Harm: Responding to the Needs of Children of Problem Drug Users.* London: Advisory Council on the Misuse of Drugs.

Horton, R. (2003) 'The neglect of child neglect [Editorial].' *Lancet, 361*, 443.

Horwath, J. (ed.) (2001) *The Child's World: Assessing Children in Need.* London: Jessica Kingsley Publishers.

Horwath, J. (2007) *Child Neglect: Identification and Assessment.* Houndsmills: Palgrave Macmillan.

Horwath, J. and Morrison, T. (2001) 'Assessment of Parental Motivation to Change.' In J. Horwath (ed.) *The Child's World: Assessing Children in Need.* London: Jessica Kingsley Publishers.

Howe, D. (2005) *Child Abuse and Neglect: Attachment, Development and Intervention.* London: Palgrave Macmillan.

Howe, D. (2008) *The Emotionally Intelligent Social Worker* Houndsmills: Palgrave Macmillan.

Howe, D. Brandon, M., Hinings, D. and Schofield, G. (1999) *Attachment Theory, Shild Maltreatment and Family Support.* London: Macmillan Press.

Hultman, C.S., Priolo, D., Cairns, B.A., Grant, E.J., Peterson, H.D. and Meyer, A.A. (1998) 'Psychosocial forum. Return to jeopardy: The fate of pediatric burn patients who are victims of abuse and neglect… including commentary by Doctor M.' *Journal of Burn Care and Rehabilitation, 19*, 4, 367–376.

Humphreys, C., Mullender, A., Thiara, R. and Skamballis, A. (2006) 'Talking to my mum: Developing communication between mothers and children in the aftermath of domestic violence.' *Journal of Social Work, 6*, 1, 53–63.

Jaudes, P., Ekwo, E. and VanVoorhis, J. (1995) 'Association of drug abuse and child abuse.' *Child Abuse and Neglect, 19*, 1065–1075.

Kandel, D. (1975) 'Reaching the hard-to-reach: Illicit drug use among high school absentees.' *Addiction Research, 1*, 4, 465–480.

Kantor, G.K., Holt, M.K., Mebert, C.J., Straus, M.A., Drach, K.M., Ricci, L.R., *et al.* (2004) 'Development and preliminary psychometric properties of the Multidimensional Neglectful Behavior Scale-Child Report.' *Child Maltreatment, 9*, 4, 409–428.

Kellogg, N. (2005) 'Oral and dental aspects of child abuse and neglect. Clinical report.' *Journal of the American Academy of Pediatrics, 116*, 6, 1565–1568.

Kelly, M., Stewart, E., Morgan, A., Killoran, A., Fischer, A., Threlfall, A., *et al.* (2009) 'A conceptual framework for public health: NICE's emerging approach.' *Public Health, 123*, e14-e20.

Kennedy, M. and Wonnacott, J. (2005) 'Neglect of Disabled Children.' In J. Taylor and B. Daniel (eds) *Child Neglect: Practice Issues for Health and Social Care.* London: Jessica Kingsley Publishers.

Kroll, B. and Taylor, A. (2001) *Parental Substance Misuse and Child Welfare.* London: Jessica Kingsley Publishers.

Kumpfer, K.L. and Tait, C. (2000) *Family Skills Training for Parents and Children.* Washington DC: U.S. Department of Justice: Office of Juvenile and Delinquency Prevention.

Lagerberg, D. (2004) 'A descriptive survey of Swedish child health nurses' awareness of abuse and neglect. II. Characteristics of the children.' *Acta Paediatrica, 93*, 5, 692–701.

Laskey, L. (2008) 'Training to Safeguard: The Australian Experience.' In M. Baginsky (ed.) *Safeguarding Children and Schools*. London: Jessica Kingsley Publishers.

Leeb, R.T., Paulozzzi, L., Melanson, C., Simon, T. and Arias, I. (2008) *Child Maltreatment Surveillance. Uniform Definitions for Public Health and Recommended Data Elements*. Atlanta, GA: Centers for Disease Control and Prevention.

Lewin, D. and Herron, H. (2007) 'Signs, symptoms and risk factors: Health visitors' perspectives of child neglect.' *Child Abuse Review, 16*, 93–107.

Ling, M.S. and Luker, K.A. (2000) 'Protecting children: Intuition and awareness in the work of health visitors.' *Journal of Advanced Nursing, 32*, 3, 572–579.

Lord Laming (2003) *The Victoria Climbié Inquiry*. London: HMSO.

Lowe, R. (2007) *Facing the Future: A Review of the Role of Health Visotrs*. London: Department of Health.

Luthar, S. (2005) 'Resilience in Development: A Synthesis of Research across Five Decades.' In D. Cicchetti and D.J. Cohen (eds) *Development Psychopathology: Risk, Disorder and Adaptation* (2nd ed., Vol. 3). New York, NY: Wiley.

Macdonald, G. (2001) *Effective Interventions for Child Abuse and Neglect: An Evidence-Based Approach to Planning and Evaluating Interventions*. Chichester: John Wiley.

Macdonald, G. (2005) 'Intervening with Neglect.' In J. Taylor and B. Daniel (eds) *Child Neglect: Practice Issues for Health and Social Care*. London: Jessica Kingsley Publishers.

Macdonald, J. and Lugton, J. (2006) 'Helping parents to understand and communicate with their babies from birth: An evaluation of an antenatal VIG teaching session.' Available at www.dundee.ac.uk/eswce/news/2009/vigconference.htm, accessed on 16 June 2011.

MacMillan, H., Wathen, C.J., Barlow, J., Fergusson, D.M., Levanthal, J.M. and Taussig, H.N. (2009) 'Interventions to prevent child maltreatment and associated impairment.' *Lancet, 373*, 250–266.

Maggiolo, C.E. (1998) *Defining the Unknown – Neglect*. USA; New-York: US Department of Education.

Maiter, S., Alaggia, R. and Trocme, N. (2004) 'Perceptions of child maltreatment by parents from the Indian subcontinent: challenging myths about culturally based abusive parenting practices.' *Child Maltreatment, 9*, 3, 309–324.

Masten, A. (1994) 'Resilience in Individual Development.' In M.C. Wang and E.W. Gordon (eds) *Educational Resilience in Inner-City America*. Hillsdale, N.J.: Erlbaum.

Matthews, J. (2010) *Melting the Iceberg of Scotland's Drug Problem. Report of the Independent Enquiry*. Glasgow: University of Glasgow.

May-Chahal, C. and Cawson, P. (2005) 'Measuring child maltreatment in the United Kingdom: A study of the prevalence of child abuse and neglect.' *Child Abuse and Neglect, 29*, 9, 969–984.

McAuley, C., Pecora, P.J. and Rose, W. (2006) *Enhancing the Well-being of Children and Families through Effective Intervention.* London: Jessica Kingsley Publishers.

McGuigan, W.M. and Pratt, C.C. (2001) 'The predictive impact of domestic violence on three types of child maltreatment.' *Child Abuse and Neglect, 25*, 7, 869–883.

McIntosh, E., Barlow, J., Davis, H. and Stewart-Brown, S. (2009) 'Economic evaluation of an intensive home visiting programme for vulnerable families: A cost-effectiveness analysis of a public health intervention.' *Journal of Public Health, 31*, 423–433.

McKeganey, N., Barnard, M. and McIntosh, J. (2002) 'Paying the price for their parents' addiction: Meeting the needs of the children of drug-using parents.' *Drugs: Education, Prevention and Policy, 9*, 3, 233–246.

Mikton, C. and Butchart, A. (2009) 'Child maltreatment prevention: A systematic review of reviews.' *Bulletin of the World Health Organization, 87*, 353–361.

Milner, J. (1986) *The Child Abuse Potential Inventory: Manual* (2nd Edition). Webster, NC: Psytec Corporation.

Mitchell, L.M., Turbiville, V. and Turnbull, H.R., III. (1999) 'Reporting abuse and neglect of children with disabilities: Early childhood service providers' views.' *Infants and Young Children, 11*, 3, 19–26.

Montgomery, P., Gardner, F., Bjornstad, G. and Ramchandani, P. (2009) *Systematic Reviews Of Interventions Following Physical Abuse: Helping Practitioners and Expert Witnesses Improve The Outcomes Of Child Abuse* (*Research Briefing*). London: Department for Education.

Moran, P. (2009) *Neglect: Research: Evidence to Inform Practice.* London: Action for Children.

Moran, P., Ghate, D. and van der Merwe, A. (2004) *What Works in Parenting Support? An International Review of Literature.* London: DfES.

Mostyn, L.W. o. (1996) *Childhood Matters: Report of the National Commission of Inquiry into the Prevention of Child Abuse* (Vol. 2). London: The Stationery Office.

Mullender, A., Hague, G., Iman, U., Kelly, L., Malos, E. and Regan, L. (2002) *Children's Perspectives on Domestic Violence.* London: Sage.

Nair, P., Black, M.M., Schuler, M., Keane, V., Snow, L., Rigney, B.A., *et al.* (1997) 'Risk factors for disruption in primary caregiving among infants of substance abusing women.' *Child Abuse and Neglect, 21*, 11, 1039–1051.

Nair, P., Schuler, M.E., Black, M.M., Kettinger, L. and Harrington, D. (2003) 'Cumulative environmental risk in substance abusing women: Early intervention, parenting stress, child abuse potential and child development.' *Child Abuse and Neglect, 27*, 9, 997–1017.

Narayan, A.P., Socolar, R.R.S. and St Claire, K. (2006) 'Pediatric residency training in child abuse and neglect in the United States.' *Pediatrics, 117*, 6, 2215–2221.

National Collaborating Centre for Women's and Children's Health (2009) *When to Suspect Child Maltreatment: Clinical Guidline.* London: RCOG Press.

National Evaluation of Sure Start (2005) *Early Impacts of Sure Start Local Programmes on Children and Families.* Available at www.ness.bbk.ac.uk, accessed on 27 January 2011.

National Evaluation of Sure Start (2008) *The Impact of Sure Start Local Programmes on Three Year olds and their Families.* London: HMSO.

National Implementation Team in England (2010) *Multidimensional Treatment Foster Care: Annual Project Report.* Available at www.mtfce.org.uk, accessed 26 May 2011.

Newman, T. (2004) *What Works in Building Resilience.* London: Barnardo's.

NSPCC (2011) Help and Advice (Publication). Available at www.nspcc.org.uk/help-and-advice/worried-about-a-child/the-nspcc-helpline/using-the-nspcc-helpline-hub_wdh72253.html, accessed on 8 January 2011.

Ofsted (2010) *Learning Lessons from Serious Case Reviews: Interim Report 2009–10.* London: Ofsted.

Ogilvie-Whyte, S. (2006) *A Review of Evidence about the Impact of Education and Training in Child Care and Protection on Practice and Client Outcomes.* Dundee: Scottish Institute for Excellence in Social Work Education.

Ondersma, S.J. (2002) 'Predictors of neglect within low-SES families: The importance of substance abuse.' *American Journal of Orthopsychiatry, 72*, 3, 383–391.

Paavilainen, E., Astedt-Kurki, P. and Paunonen, M. (2000) 'School nurses' operational modes and ways of collaborating in caring for child abusing families in Finland.' *Journal of Clinical Nursing, 9*, 5, 742–750.

Paavilainen, E., Merikanto, J., Astedt-Kurki, P., Laippala, P., Tammentie, T. and Paunonen-Ilmonen, M. (2002) 'Identification of child maltreatment while caring for them in a university hospital.' *International Journal of Nursing Studies, 39*, 3, 287–294.

Paavilainen, E. and Tarkka, M. (2003) 'Definition and identification of child abuse by Finnish public health nurses.' *Public Health Nursing, 20*, 1, 49–55.

Reading, R., Bissell, S., Goldhagen, J., Harwin, J., Masson, J., Moynihan, S., *et al.* (2009) 'Promotion of children's rights and prevention of child maltreatment.' *The Lancet, 373*, 332–343.

Reder, P. and Duncan, S. (1995) 'The Meaning of the Child.' In P. Reder and C. Lucey (eds), *Assessment of Parenting: Psychiatric and Psychological Contributions.* London and New York, NY: Routledge.

Reder, P., Duncan, S. and Gray, M. (1993) *Beyond Blame: Child Abuse Tragedies Revisited.* London: Routledge.

Reder, P. and Lucey, C. (1995) 'Significant issues in the assessment of parenting.' In P. Reder and C. Lucey (eds), *Assessment of Parenting: Psychiatric and Psychological Contributions.* London: Routledge.

Rose, S.J. and Meezan, W. (1995) 'Child neglect: A study of the perceptions of mothers and child welfare workers.' *Children and Youth Services Review, 17,* 4, 471–486.

Rose, S.J. and Meezan, W. (1996) 'Variations in perceptions of child neglect.' *Child Welfare Journal, 75,* 2, 139–160.

Rose, S.J. and Selwyn, J. (2000) 'Child neglect: An English perspective.' *International Social Work, 43,* 2, 179–192.

Rubin, D., O'Reilly, A., Luan, X. and Localio, R. (2007) 'The impact of placement instability on behavioral well-being for children in foster care.' *Pediatrics, 119,* 336–344.

Rutter, M. (1987) 'Psychosocial resilience and protective mechanisms.' *American Journal of Orthopsychiatry, 57,* 316–331.

Sanders, M., Pidgeon, A., Gravestock, F., Connors, M.D., Brown, S. and Young R.W. (2004) 'Does parental attributional retraining and anger management enhance the effects of the Triple P – Positive Parenting Program with parents at risk of child maltreatment?' *Behavior Therapy, 35,* 3, 513–535.

Scannapieco, M. and Connell-Carrick, K. (2003) 'Families in poverty: Those who maltreat their infants and toddlers and those who do not.' *Journal of Family Social Work, 7,* 3, 49–70.

Scannapieco, M. and Connell-Carrick, K. (2005) 'Focus on the First Years: Correlates of substantiation of child maltreatment for families with children 0 to 4.' *Children and Youth Services Review 27,* 1307–1323.

Scott, D. (2009) *A Public Health Approach to Child Protection* [*seminar report*]. Stirling: Scottish Child Care and Protection Network.

Scott, D. (2010) 'Child Abuse and Neglect: Is Prevention Possible? Yes! [seminar].' *Pacific Association of Child Abuse and Neglect, Australia,* January.

Scott, D. and Taylor, J. (2010) 'Towards a public health approach in protecting and nurturing children: From metaphor to method [Conference Report].' *ISPCAN XVIII International Conference, Honolulu, Hawaii,* 26–29 September.

Scott, K. (2008) 'Caring Dads [online].' Available at www.caringdadsprogram.com, accessed on 6 April 2010.

Scott, K. and Crooks, C.V. (2004) 'Effecting change in maltreating fathers: Critical principles for intervention planning.' *Clinical Psychology, 11,* 95–111.

Scottish Executive (2002) *'It's Everyone's Job to Make Sure I'm Alright.' Report of the Child Protection Audit and Review.* Edinburgh: The Scottish Executive.

Scottish Executive (2004) *The Children's Charter.* Edinburgh: The Scottish Executive.

Scottish Executive (2005) *Getting it Right for Every Child: Proposals for Action.* Edinburgh: Scottish Executive.

Scottish Government (2008) '*A Guide to Getting it Right for Every Child.*' Edinburgh: Scottish Government.

Scottish Government (2009) 'Getting it Right for Every Child – Overview [online].' Available at www.scotland.gov.uk/Topics/People/Young-People/childrensservices/girfec/programme-overview, accessed on 5 December 2010.

Scottish Government (2010a) *National Guidance for Child Protection in Scotland.* Edinburgh: Scottish Government.

Scottish Government (2010b) *All You Need to Know about Swine Flu* [online]. Available at www.scotland.gov.uk/Topics/Health/health/flu/pandemic, accessed on 28 November 2010.

Sfikas, P.M. (1999) 'Dentistry and the law. Reporting abuse and neglect.' *Journal of the American Dental Association: JADA, 130,* 12, 1797–1799.

Sheehan, R. (2004) 'Partnership in mental health and child welfare: Social work responses to children living with parental mental illness.' *Social Work in Health Care, 39,* 3/4, 309–324.

Smith, M.G. and Fong, R. (2004) *The Children of Neglect: When No One Cares.* New York, NY and Hove: Brunner-Routledge.

Stagner, M.W. and Lansing, J. (2009) 'Progress towards a prevention perspective.' *Future of Children, 19,* 2, 19–38.

Stein, M., Rees, G., Hicks, L. and Gorin, S. (2009) *Neglected Adolescents: Literature Review: Research Brief, DCSF-RBX-09-04.* London: Department for Children, Schools and Families.

Stevenson, O. (1998) *Neglected Children: Issues and Dilemmas.* Oxford: Blackwell.

Stevenson, O. (2007) *Neglected Children and Their Families.* Oxford: Blackwell.

Stradling, B., MacNeil, M. and Berry, H. (2009) *Changing Professional Practice and Culture to Get it Right for Every Child: An Evaluation of the Early Development Phases of Getting it Right for Every Child in Highland: 2006–2009.* Edinburgh: Scottish Government.

Sullivan, P.M. and Knutson, J.F. (2000) 'Maltreatment and disabilities: A population based epidemiological study.' *Child Abuse and Neglect, 24,* 1257–1273.

Svrivastava, O.P., Fountain, R., Ayre, P. and Stewart, J. (2003) 'The Graded Care Profile: A Measure of Care.' In M. Calder and S. Hackett (eds) *Assessment in Child Care.* Dorset: Russell House Publishing.

Tanner, K. and Turney, D. (2003) 'What do we know about child neglect? A critical review of the literature and its application to social work practice.' *Child and Family Social Work, 8,* 1, 25–34.

Tanner, K. and Turney, D. (2006) 'Therapeutic Interventions with Children who have Experienced Neglect and their Families in the UK.' In C. McAuley, P.J. Pecora and W. Rose (eds) *Enhancing the Well-being of Children and Families through Effective Intervention.* London: Jessica Kingsley Publishers.

Taylor, J. (2010) *Scoping Report: Physical Abuse in High Risk Families.* London: NSPCC.

Taylor, J., Baldwin, N. and Spencer, N. (2008) 'Predicting child abuse and neglect: Ethical, theoretical and methodological challenges.' *Journal of Clinical Nursing, 17*, 1193–1200.

Taylor, J. and Daniel, B. (eds) (2005) *Neglect: Practice Issues for Health and Social Care.* London: Jessica Kingsley Publishers.

Thoburn, J. (2009) *Effective Interventions for Complex Families where there are Concerns About, or Evidence of, A Child Suffering Significant Harm.* London: Centre for Excellence and Outcomes for Children (C4EO).

Thomas, N., Stainton, T., Jackson, S., Yee Cheung, W., Doubtfire, S. and Webb, A. (2003) "Your friends don't understand": Invisibility and unmet need in the lives of "young carers".' *Child and Family Social Work, 8*, 35–46.

Thyen, U., Leventhal, J.M., Yazdgerdi, S.R. and Perrin, J.M. (1997) 'Concerns about Child Maltreatment in Hospitalized Children.' *Child Abuse and Neglect: The International Journal, 21*, 2, 187–198.

Tunstill, J. (2007) *Volunteers in Child Protection: A study and evaluation of CSV's pilot projects in Sunderland and Bromley.* London: Community Service Volunteers (CSV).

Tunstill, J. and Aldgate, J. (2000) *Services for Children in Need: From Policy to Practice.* London: The Stationery Office.

Turney, D. (2005) 'Who cares? The role of mothers in cases of child neglect.' In J. Taylor and B. Daniel (eds) *Child Neglect: Practice Issues for Health and Social Care.* London: Jessica Kingsley Publishers.

Twardosz, S. and Lutzker, J.R. (2010) 'Child maltreatment and the developing brain: A review of neuroscience perspectives.' *Aggression and Violent Behavior, 15*, 1, 59–68.

Udwin, O. (1983) 'Imaginative play training as an intervention method with institutionalised pre-school children. ' *British Journal of Educational Psychology, 53*, 32–39.

United Nations (1989) *United Nations Convention on the Rights of the Child.* New York, NY: General Assembly of the United Nations.

Velleman, R. and Orford, J. (1999) *Risk and Resilience: Adults Who Were the Children of Problem Drinkers.* Amsterdam, the Netherlands: Harwood Academic Publishers.

Vincent, S. and Daniel, B. (2004) 'An analysis of children and young people's calls to ChildLine about abuse and neglect: A study for the Scottish child protection review.' *Child Abuse Review, 13*, 2, 158–171.

Violence Against Women Scotland (2009) CEDAR Project. Available from www.vawpreventionscotland.org.uk/directory/stirling/cedar-project, accessed on 27 January 2011.

Weavers, I.C.G. (2009) 'Shaping adult phenotypes through early life environments.' *Birth Defects Research (Part C), 87*, 314–326.

Webster, S.W., O'Toole, R., O'Toole, A.W. and Lucal, B. (2005) 'Overreporting and underreporting of child abuse: Teachers' use of professional discretion.' *Child Abuse and Neglect, 29,* 1281–1296

Wilding, J. and Thoburn, J. (1997) 'Family support plans for neglected and emotionally maltreated children.' *Child Abuse Review, 6,* 5, 343–356.

Wright, C. and Birks, E. (2000a) 'Risk factors for failure to thrive: a population-based survey.' *Child: Care, Health and Development, 26,* 1, 5–16.

Wright, C. and Birks, E. (2000b) 'Risk factors for failure to thrive: A population-based survey.' *Child: Care, Health and Development, 26,* 1, 5–16.

Zeanah, C., Larrieu, J.A., Heller, S.S., Valliere, J., Hinshaw-Fuselier, S., Aoki, Y., *et al.* (2001) 'Evaluation of a preventive intervention for maltreated infants and toddlers in foster care.' *Journal of the American Academy of Child and Adolescent Psychiatry, 40,* 214–221.

Subject Index

Author Index